The No-Nonsense Guide to
Cosmetic Surgery

by Sheldon Rothfleisch, M.D.

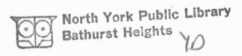
Publishers · GROSSET & DUNLAP · New York
A FILMWAYS COMPANY

Contents

Preface

This book was not written to extol the benefits of plastic surgery. We have assumed that the reader is already sold on the concept of cosmetic surgery but is searching for more specific information. Our purpose, then, is to inform you in a concise manner and in understandable terms.

The surgical procedures most commonly requested are presented here with information regarding cost range, basic surgical technique, length of hospital stay and recuperation period, and potential complications. This information is meant to be a guide to you, the patient, prior to, or following, a consultation with a reputable plastic surgeon.

It should be emphasized that the specific surgical techniques described in this book are the preference of the author, and are certainly not intended to be presented as the only acceptable techniques for performing each procedure. You should be guided by your own surgeon's choice of the exact techniques to be used in any specific operation.

At the outset, a word should be said regarding the selection of a surgeon. We suggest that you seek a Board-certified plastic surgeon. Board certification is obtained on the successful completion of a comprehensive examination in the area of specialization. This ensures that you are being cared for by a physician who has completed several years of general surgical training, followed by two to three years of plastic surgical training.

Aside from technical know-how, whenever you choose a doctor there still remains that elusive and intangible aesthetic sense, which is so important, but also subjective. Here you do best to rely on recommendations based on skillful past performance. These recommendations may come from a trusted family physician or general surgeon, your local medical society, or perhaps a satisfied friend. In many situations, the results of a plastic surgeon's work are highly visible. Finally, your choice should be based on your impressions after you have had your consultation. Your surgeon should have discussed the procedure with you in some detail, answered all reasonable questions, and been frank about cost, including the perhaps unanticipated costs of hospitalization and anesthesia. All these matters should be weighed carefully before you go ahead with the procedure.

THE
FACE

Face Lift (Rhytidectomy)

Purpose: To correct the laxity of the skin caused by aging.

Overview: Unfortunately, in no other part of the body is aging more apparent than in the face. Exposure to ultraviolet light accelerates the aging process by altering the connective tissue (the supporting fibers) of the skin. The contribution of sunlight to the skin's aging varies in individuals, depending upon the amount of exposure and the skin pigmentation. Deeper complexioned people are less susceptible than the fair-skinned to the effects of ultraviolet light. Nevertheless, what results to varying degrees as people age is wrinkling, looseness of skin texture, loss of skin elasticity, patchy areas of increased or decreased pigmentation, excessive dryness, excessive glossiness of skin surface, and an increasing number of skin tumors.

If these distressing symptoms of aging were not enough, the effects of gravity and muscular action are responsible for horizontal and vertical frown lines on the forehead, crow's feet at the corners of the eyelids, midline forehead wrinkles, nose-to-lip fold wrinkles, jowls, and fine wrinkles about the mouth. All are the result of complex biochemical and biomechanical processes, the mechanisms of which are not completely understood, and all contribute to the look of aging.

Patients who seek surgery in order to alter the appearance of an aging face generally fit into one of several groups. One group consists of people in their late thirties, usually women with slightly sagging jowls and some wrinkling. These patients often desire a face lift in order to compete socially with younger women.

Working women in their forties and early fifties who seek surgery often do so in order to maintain their position in in the job market. Men in the same age group may be similarly motivated.

Widowed or divorced persons may seek facial surgery for an emotional lift. Some may be motivated by a desire to establish personal relationships with younger prospective partners.

Not everyone who wishes to have a face lift is a suitable surgical candidate. No one can trim ten to twenty years off your appearance or make you resemble your school yearbook photograph; a more realistic goal is to appear less tired and harried and in general more attractive. Nor can facial surgery patch up your ailing marriage or assure your promotion at work. And if you are very overweight, you should be discouraged from seeking surgery until weight reduction has been achieved and maintained for at least six months if you want satisfactory results.

Time and Place: This procedure is most commonly performed in a hospital, although it can be done in a well-equipped office or clinic, with some reduction in overall cost to you. Anesthesia may be local or general; this should be discussed with your surgeon preoperatively. The physician's fee for general anesthesia adds to the cost of the surgery.

Preparation: An antiseptic scrub (Betadine® or Phisohex®) will be used on your face and hair one to several days prior to surgery.

On the day of the operation, small areas of scalp hair are shaved at sites to be used for surgical incision. (These scars are usually not noticeable postoperatively.) You can braid your hair or get it to lie flat against your scalp by using K-Y jelly. If the procedure is to be done under local anesthesia, you will be given sedation two hours and one hour prior to surgery. Generally the medications given are narcotics and barbiturates.

Procedure: Incisions are made in the hairline at the temple and are extended downward along the crease in front of the ear (preauricular crease), around the lobule of the ear to the area behind the ear, and on to the upper neck. If the surgery is being performed under local anesthesia, all incision sites are preinjected. By careful dissection, the facial skin (flaps) are elevated toward the crease of the mouth (nasolabial fold) and downward to the neck. Whatever bleeding occurs is controlled. After any pockets of fat are removed, tucking sutures are placed along the gravity lines. "Plication" is the term used to describe this procedure. Muscle plication (tightening) is also performed on the neck muscles to create a smooth, wrinkle-free neck. When the plications are completed, the skin is allowed to drape over the incision lines, and any excess skin is removed, but without creating skin tension. Drains are seldom needed, and closure is accomplished by fine suturing. Dressings consist of a medicated gauze that is positioned along the suture lines and applied with moderate compression on the facial flaps. These dressings are usually removed after twenty-four hours, and the area is redressed. All dressings are removed in seventy-two hours or less. On the fifth day after surgery, all visible sutures are removed; the remaining stay sutures are taken out on the tenth day.

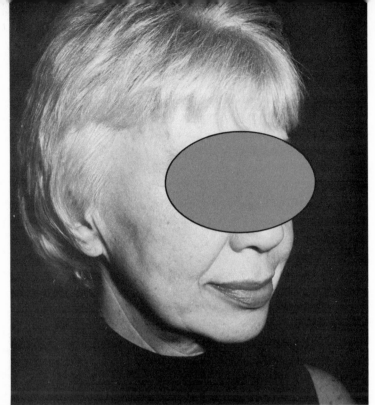

Face Lift—pre-op

Face Lift—pre-op, neck

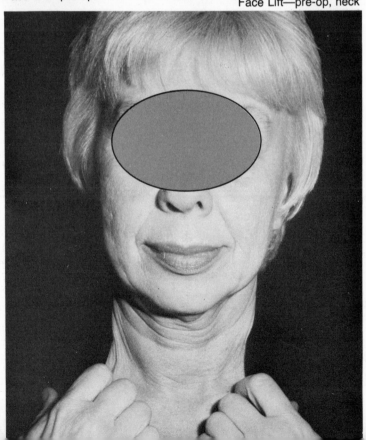

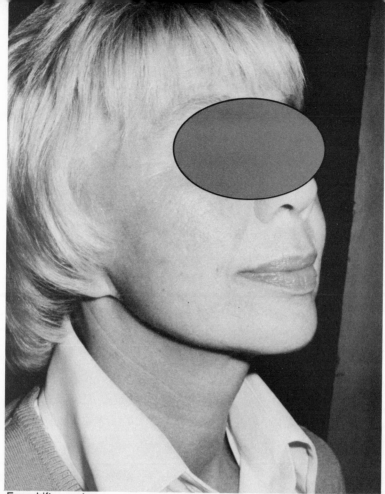

Face Lift—post-op

Face Lift—post-op, neck

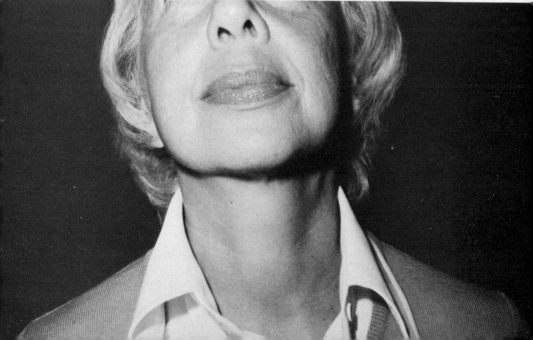

Pain and Discomfort: If you are like most patients, you can expect to be pain-free in twenty-four to forty-eight hours. Prolonged pain or severe acute pain may signal a complication.

Aftereffects: Many patients have small black-and-blue areas (ecchymoses), and swelling may last several days to a week. Large areas of black-and-blue marks may be a sign of impending skin damage and should be investigated.

A feeling of "tightness" is to be expected and may persist for several weeks. If you lie with your head elevated, this helps to reduce swelling. Most patients are ambulatory with no restrictions after one or two days.

The dressings are usually inspected or even changed within twenty-four hours. Sutures placed in front of the ears are removed within five days; the remaining sutures are taken out seven to ten days later. You may shampoo your hair once the sutures are removed, but using makeup is discouraged for about two weeks.

Complications: Sensory losses generally occur and can last a few weeks or a few months. On occasion, loss of sensation evidenced by numbness may be permanent. Do not be upset if you have some swelling and ecchymosis; almost all patients experience this. Small subcutaneous collections of blood and serum are usually absorbed spontaneously, but large collections threaten the viability of the overlying skin and require prompt drainage. Excessive pain should be reported; this may herald the onset of a large collection of blood.

Occasionally, small areas of skin are lost, but these almost always heal uneventfully.

A serious complication is injury to a segment of the facial nerve resulting in segmental paralysis of the facial musculature with subsequent facial asymmetry. Fortunately, this type of injury rarely occurs.

Cost: Varies from $1,500–$6,000.

Nose Reconstruction
(Rhinoplasty)

Purpose: To achieve an aesthetically pleasing shape and contour of the nose.

Overview: Rhinoplasty is a procedure by which structural alterations are made in the supporting tissues of the nose. This surgery is performed intranasally (inside the nose) and therefore yields no external scars. Portions of bone, cartilage, and soft tissue are trimmed from the nose, and the supporting bone is fractured and repositioned. The final result is a composite of these structural alterations in combination with the texture of the skin that surfaces it.

A well-executed procedure sometimes yields disappointing results because of the patient's innate capacity for healing. The most favorable results are achieved with patients in their twenties. At either end of the age spectrum, results may be less satisfying. For example, a teenager with thick oily skin complicated by active acne can present a problem because of the poor draping ability of this unyielding skin. In older people, the inelastic nature of the skin can also result in poor draping with thickness in the tip of the nose.

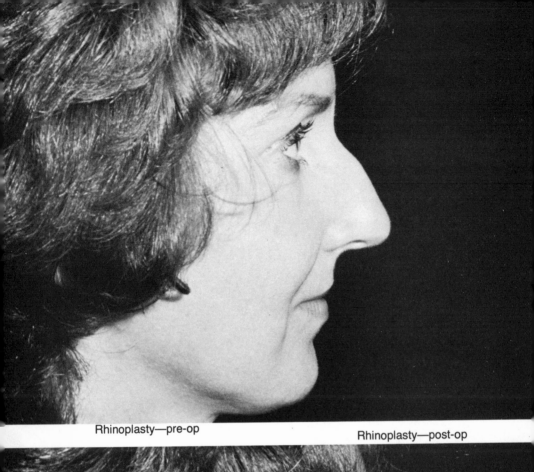

Rhinoplasty—pre-op

Rhinoplasty—post-op

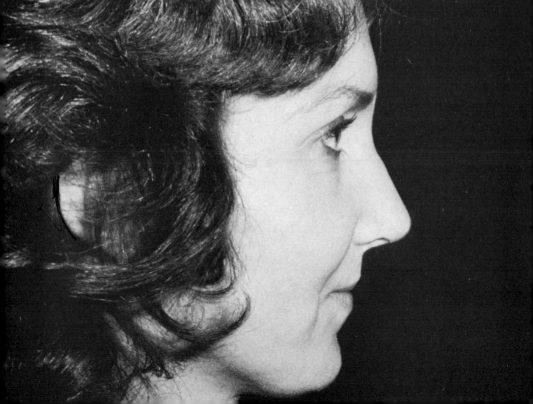

It is unrealistic to expect a surgeon to duplicate the photograph of a particular celebrity. Most cosmetic surgeons have a good sense of aesthetics and try to fashion a nose that will suit your general facial structure. On occasion, a surgeon may even recommend a recontouring of a patient's chin in order to balance the facial profile. (This will be discussed in the chapter on chin implants.)

Time and Place: This procedure is generally performed in a hospital under local or general anesthesia. The operation takes about one and one-half hours, and the patient is hospitalized from two to three days.

Preparation: Your face will be cleansed with an antiseptic scrub on the night prior to surgery. Preoperative sedation will be administered just before surgery if the procedure is to be done under local anesthesia. In the operating suite, your face will again be scrubbed and prepped, and the nasal vibrissae (hairs) will be clipped.

Procedure: After the nose is packed (to prevent aspiration of blood), the nasal tip, bridge, and columella are injected with a local anesthetic. The area beneath the eyes (infraorbital region) is also injected. Incisions are made inside the nose. The entire dorsum (upper surface) of the nose is elevated. The cartilage tip is remodeled. The dorsal septal cartilage is then trimmed; and the bony hump of the nose is sawed, chiseled, or rasped off. A medial and lateral bone fracture is performed, and the fractured nasal bones are moved inward to narrow the nasal bridge. Excess mucosal lining is trimmed from within the nose, after which the final rasping and trimming of the cartilage is performed. Openings in the nose tip are sewn up. Packing is usually placed within the nose to support the tip and the septum. A splint is applied to the dorsum of the nose after appropriate padding is in place. The splint may be made of plaster, metal, or a dental compound. It generally remains in place two to six days, although in some cases it may be left on for two weeks.

Pain and Discomfort: Moderate discomfort may require pain medication for twenty-four hours after your operation. Nasal packing can add to your discomfort, and these often must remain in place for three to four days.

Aftereffects and Complications: Facial blemishes, pigment rings around the eyes, acne scars, dilated capillaries, asymmetrical nostrils, septal perforations, disfigurements about the mouth, and certain skin conditions (e.g., smooth and oily, rough and dry) can influence the results.

Hemorrhage and hematoma can occur following surgery. The most frequent site of hemorrhage is the nasal septum and second most frequent is the nasal tip. Nasal tip hemorrhage may result in thickening and distortion in the months following surgery. Septal hematoma can lead to perforation and infection of the septum which in turn may result in loss of nasal support.

Delayed hemorrhage is possible as late as ten to fourteen days postoperatively. This can be prevented by avoiding blowing the nose or postoperative manipulation. In addition, you should be cautioned against bending, which increases intracranial and intranasal pressure; straining unduly; or performing excessively active exercise.

Possible Residual Deformities: The overwhelming majority of patients do not experience any residual deformities. Possibly 5 percent of patients may require secondary rhinoplasty as a result of residual deformities, which include:

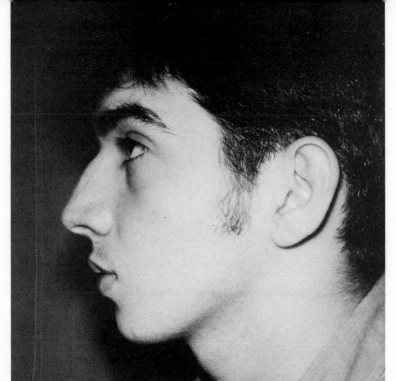

Rhinoplasty—pre-op

Rhinoplasty—post-op

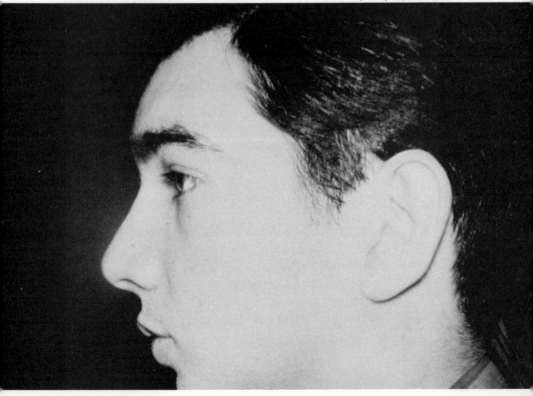

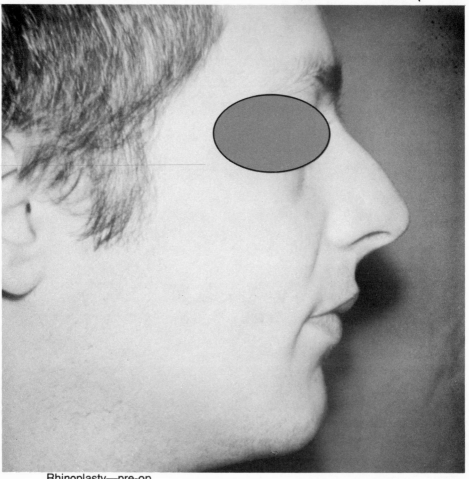

Rhinoplasty—pre-op

1. Excessive scar contraction of the intranasal incision, which can lead to a narrowing of the nostril.
2. "Parrot beak" or "Polly beak" formation, which can be the result of excessive proliferation of scar tissue in the nasal tip or excess cartilage on the dorsum.
3. Residual hump deformity of the dorsum of the nose.
4. A ski-jump (Bob Hope or saddle) nose.
5. Asymmetry of the nose caused by uneven healing of the fractured bones.
6. Spreading of the nasal bones, which may result from callus formation causing separation of the nasal bones.

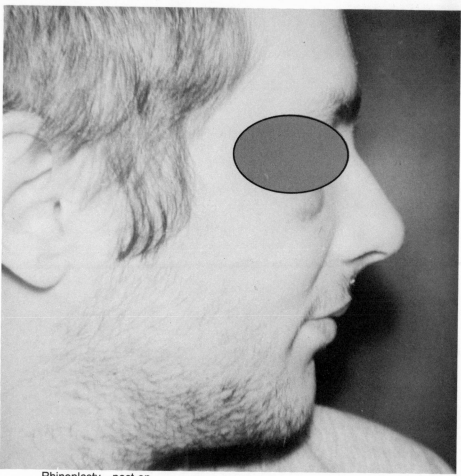

Rhinoplasty—post-op

7. Collapsed, depressed, pinched, dropped, or deviated tip.
8. Hanging columella, usually associated with a dropped tip.

Cost: The range is $1,000–$3,000. Check with your insurance company. Coverage may be available if you are suffering from a septal deformity that requires correction. Naturally, the extent of coverage varies with the quality of the insurance policy.

Correction of Eyelid Changes (Blepharoplasty)

Purpose: To correct baggy eyelids.

Overview: Bagginess about the eyes is most commonly associated with the aging process. Nevertheless, several conditions that may respond to conservative medical measures can cause eyelid changes, so you should see your medical doctor before considering a blepharoplasty. These conditions include changes resulting from kidney disease, heart failure, lung disease, and certain endocrine (glandular) disorders. Bagginess about the eyes can also be allergic or infectious in nature, and if so, should be treated accordingly. Finally, one may, on rare occasions, see young persons in whom the muscles about the eyes have undergone enlargement.

The earliest sign of eyelid changes caused by aging is sagging of the upper eyelid. This may be followed by sagging of the lower lid. If these changes are severe, they can lead to mechanical impairment of vision. In addition to sagging, bulging (herniation) of the fat pads located beneath the lids accentuates the problem.

Time and Place: This procedure can be performed in an outpatient facility or in a hospital. Local or general anesthesia may be used. One and one-half hours of operating time are usually required.

Preparation: Your hair will be shampooed and your face scrubbed with an antiseptic solution on the evening prior to surgery. To allay anxiety, you will be given preoperative sedation one hour prior to surgery. This is particularly important when surgery is to be performed under local anesthesia.

Procedure: After the patient is well sedated, markings are made indicating the lines of incision. Injections of anesthesia containing epinephrine to reduce bleeding are made locally. If the anesthesia is general, a vasoconstrictor alone is administered. Incisions are made, and the superfluous upper-lid skin is removed; this is followed by removal of protruding orbital fat. The site is then sutured. The procedure is repeated on the lower lid, with the mouth held open in order to create maximum tension on the lower lid. After suturing, antibiotic ointment is applied. Some surgeons apply a gentle pressure dressing for twenty-four to forty-eight hours. Patients often wear dark glasses for several days after the surgery to relieve glare and reduce stare. Sutures are removed in three to five days.

Aftereffects: You may have considerable swelling and discoloration about your eyes and blood stains in the white (sclera) of the eye. These effects usually disappear within two weeks. Crinkle lines that appear on smiling are not eradicated by this procedure, a fact that should be clearly understood by anyone planning to undergo the surgery.

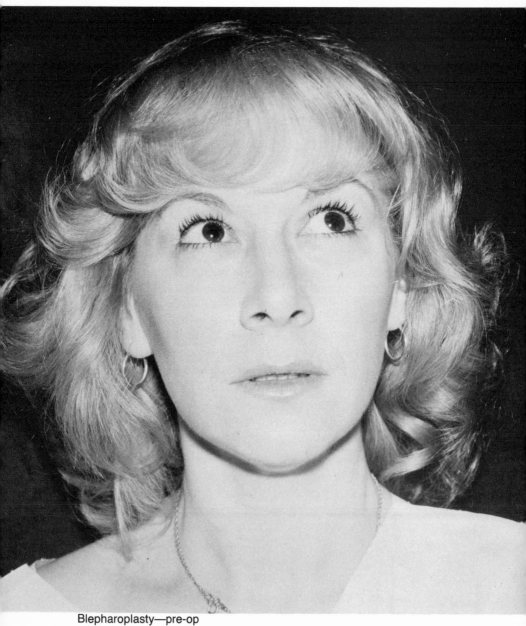

Blepharoplasty—pre-op

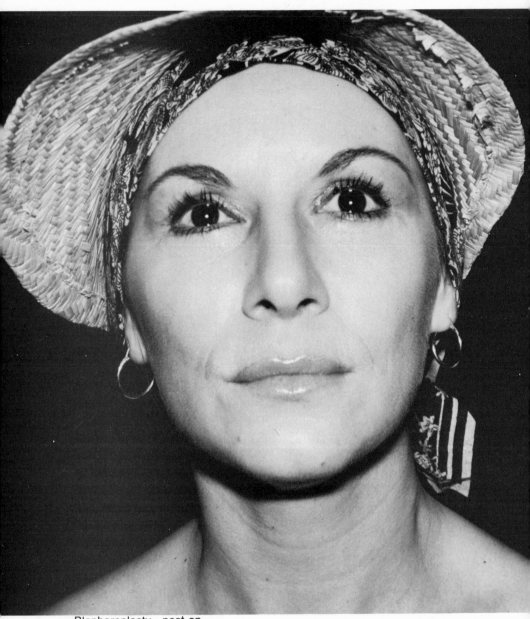

Blepharoplasty—post-op

Complications: Inclusion cysts may develop along the suture line. Occasionally the scars become thick, but they tend to settle down with time. Suture abscesses may develop, but these generally clear once the stitches are removed. Corneal abrasion and direct injury to the globe of the eye is rare.

Ectropian of the lower lid (a pulling down of the lower lid that results in exposure of the sclera) is a more serious complication. This can develop temporarily after surgery because of loss of tone. If the contour is not resolved spontaneously after several weeks, additional surgery may be required to correct this complication.

The most severe and, fortunately, rare complication is retrobulbar hemorrhage leading to blindness.

Despite the possible complications, blepharoplasty is generally an effective and safe procedure.

Cost: Varies from $750–$2,000.

Brow Lift

Purpose: To correct forehead wrinkles and drooping of the upper eyelids.

Overview: Three basic muscle groups are responsible for expression of the forehead that can produce wrinkling. The major muscle of the forehead, the frontalis, permits vertical movement, which can lead to horizontal wrinkles. Vertical frown lines are produced by the action of two muscles called corrugators. Horizontal wrinkles over the roof of the nose (known as the glabella) are produced by the procerus muscle. Eliminating these muscular actions results in the elimination of frown lines.

When the brow is located below the bony rim above the eye (the supraorbital rim) it causes bulging and drooping of the upper eyelid. A direct brow lift can alleviate this problem.

There are several techniques for performing a brow, or forehead, lift. Brow lifts also may be performed in conjunction with a face lift (rhytidectomy), eye lift (blepharoplasty), or nose reconstruction (rhinoplasty). Procedures for two kinds of brow lifts follow.

Time and Place: This brow lift can be done in the hospital or at a clinic with local or general anesthesia.

Preparation: Your hair will be shampooed and your face cleansed with an antiseptic solution. Your hair will be braided to permit easy access to the incision site.

Procedure for Brow, or Forehead, Lift: The incision is made from the upper part of the ear over the top of the head to the opposite ear. The forehead is elevated from the underlying bone down to the roof of the nose. Bleeding is generally minimal. Muscle segments are removed to reduce the horizontal lines caused by muscle contraction. The muscle is cut high on the forehead so that the lower half of the muscles can animate the eyebrows, thereby permitting expression. After applying some tension, excess skin is removed from the top of the head; suturing is then carried out. Drains are an option of the surgeon. Their use depends, of course, on the degree of bleeding present.

Advantages: In conjunction with a blepharoplasty, a brow lift usually gives a favorable result for the elderly patient with drooping forehead and upper lids. Unlike the direct approach, there are no easily visible scars. The surgeon has access to the dorsum of the nose, and even a rhinoplasty can be performed through the same incision site.

Disadvantages: In patients with a high hairline, the brow lift may further raise the hairline. Bald males, on whom the surgical scar cannot be hidden, are poor candidates for this procedure. The operating time required for this procedure is greater than that required for the routine Direct Brow Lift (see below).

Pain and Discomfort: For a week to ten days after the brow lift you will experience a tugging sensation, but pain and discomfort are generally minimal. Acute and severe pain may indicate a complication such as a hematoma (a collection of blood under the skin).

Complications: Unless you have a clotting disorder or high blood pressure, the risk of excessive bleeding is small. Nerve injury is a potential hazard, as is hair loss (traumatic alopecia) that results from tension on the flaps when forehead skin is brought to scalp skin.

Procedure for Direct Brow Lift: The direct brow lift is accomplished by excising an elliptical segment of skin and subcutaneous tissue in the area above the eyebrow bilaterally. The bulk of the resection is located more laterally, that is, toward the temple. This essentially lifts the lateral part of the eyebrow and upper lid, where the sagging is greatest. It also accomplishes a considerable improvement in the central portions of the upper lid. Mild to moderate degrees of upper-lid drooping can be completely corrected solely with a direct brow lift. In more severe cases, a brow lift in conjunction with a standard blepharoplasty can enhance the cosmetic result. This procedure can also be performed in conjunction with a standard face lift and in some cases may eliminate the need for upper-lid blepharoplasty.

Complications: The complications associated with a direct brow lift are limited. A potential problem is the scar that is left on the forehead. Although lying in a transverse direction, which decreases its visibility, the scar may serve as a deterrent to the direct approach.

Cost: Both procedures range from $750–$2,000.

Reshaping the Ears
(Otoplasty)

Purpose: To correct protruding or oddly contoured ears.

Overview: Protruding ears, sometimes referred to as "cup" or "lop" ears, exhibit excess cartilage, a lack of infolding of the upper portion of the ear, and an increased angle of protrusion from the scalp. The normal ear protrudes 1.7 to 2.0 centimeters from the scalp; an abnormally protruding ear exceeds this number by 0.5 to 1.5 centimeters.

There are three basic components of the abnormally protruding ear: (1) an inadequate upper-ear fold (known as the antehelical fold); (2) an excessive amount of cartilage in the cavity of the ear (excessive conchal cartilage); and (3) protrusion of the earlobe secondary to protrusion of the tail of the helix (the incurved rim of the external ear).

Because a child with protruding ears is often subjected to ridicule by his peers, corrective surgery is best performed before he starts kindergarten.

Ear deformities may be associated with urinary or kidney abnormalities, so the presence of such conditions

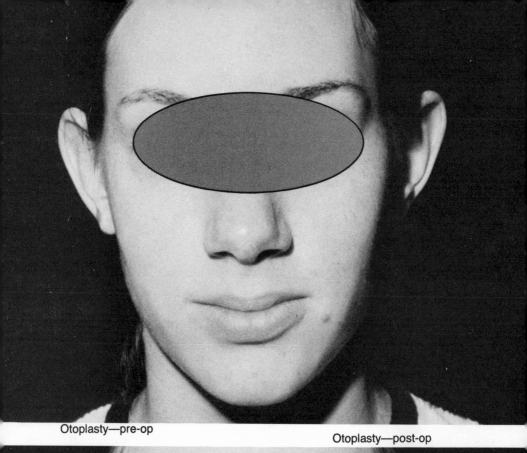

Otoplasty—pre-op

Otoplasty—post-op

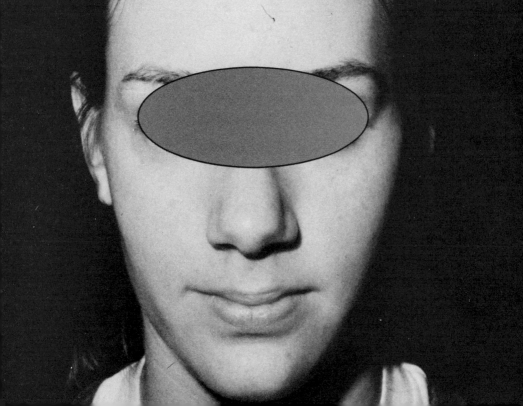

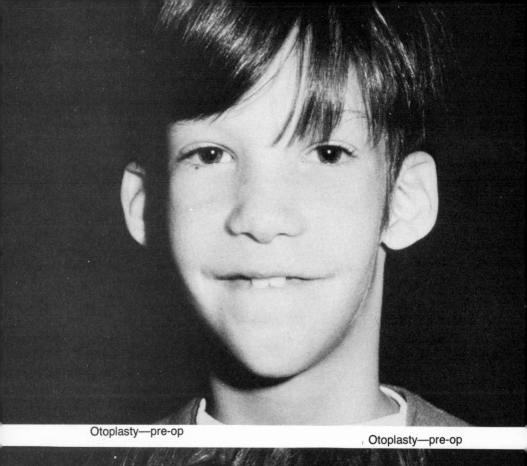

Otoplasty—pre-op

Otoplasty—pre-op

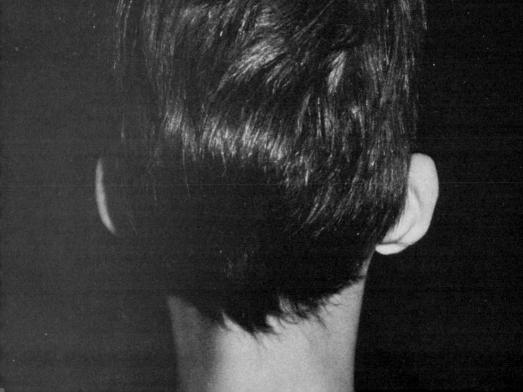

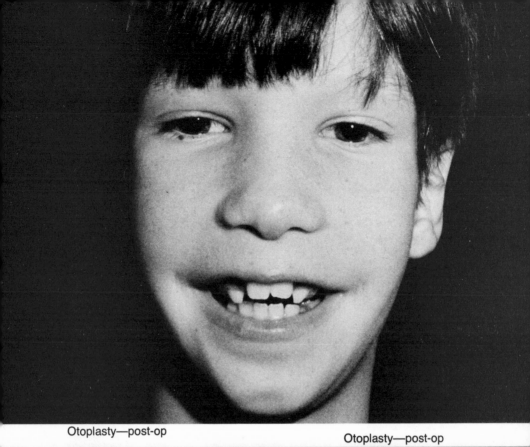

Otoplasty—post-op

Otoplasty—post-op

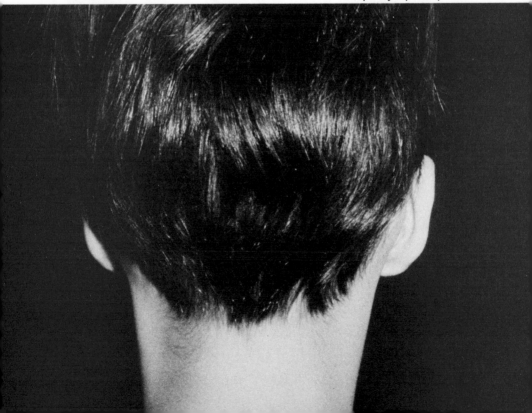

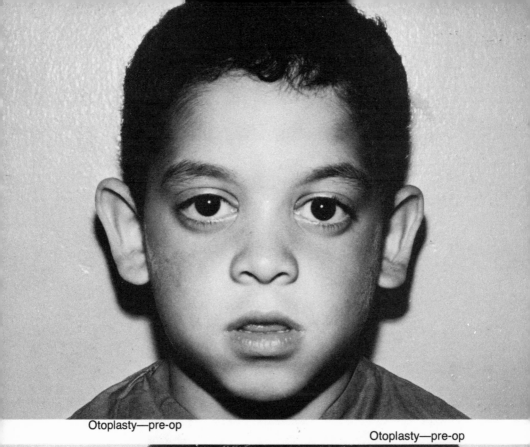

Otoplasty—pre-op

Otoplasty—pre-op

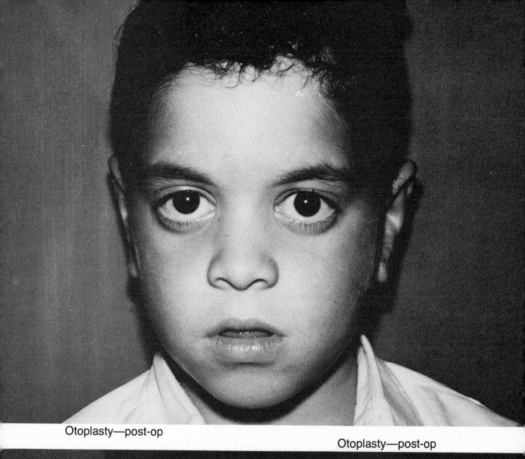

Otoplasty—post-op

Otoplasty—post-op

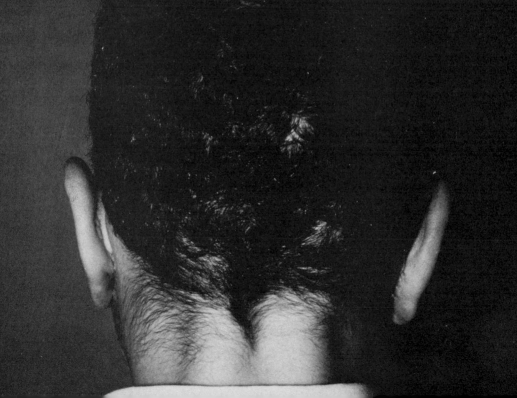

should be investigated before any cosmetic surgery is contemplated.

Time and Place: This procedure is most often performed in the hospital under general anesthesia. A well-equipped clinic may be a suitable alternative, however, and local anesthesia may be used. Operating time varies with the technique, but generally runs one and one-half hours. When hospitalized, the patient's stay averages three days.

Preparation: The patient's face and ears will be scrubbed with an antiseptic solution. Preoperative sedation will be administered.

Procedure: Incisions are made on the outer surface of the ear. The cartilage is exposed and scored (scratched), which causes the cartilage to bend in the opposite direction. Sutures are placed at appropriate points on the posterior cartilage to maintain the position established by scoring. The sutures are nonabsorbable, and their placement establishes the appropriate unfolding of the upper ear. Resection of excessive conchal cartilage is performed; if necessary, this area may be sutured to the scalp to provide further setback. The tail and lobule of the ear are trimmed to improve contour. The incisions are then closed, and molded dressings, which consist of mineral oil impregnated cotton gauze, and an ace-type bandage for compression, are applied.

The dressing is removed in about five days and a ski-type band is worn continuously for four weeks and then at night only for an additional six weeks. Sutures are removed seven to ten days after surgery.

Complications: The most serious complication is hematoma (a collection of blood). Any hematoma must be drained to prevent infection of the cartilage, which if allowed to progress would result in cauliflower ears or a similar distortion in shape. Severe and unrelenting pain postoperatively should be reported; it may be a clue to the development of a hematoma or may result from excessive pressure from the dressing.

Recurrence of the original deformity is possible as late as a year after surgery. Premature discontinuation of the headband at night can cause the deformity to reappear.

Keloids are another potential problem. These are thick scars that will mar the operation's results. Keloids are infrequently seen in Caucasian patients but are more common for blacks.

Cost: An otoplasty costs $750–$1,850.

Chin Augmentation (Mentoplasty)

Purpose: To correct a recessed chin.

Overview: Mentoplasty is a procedure in which chin projection is increased by inserting an implant, which can consist of either the patient's own tissue or alloplastic material. The prosthetic device is placed in a pocket created in front of the jaw. In microgenia, the condition this technique corrects, the jaw is functionally normal but lacks the forward projection of the chin eminence. Occasionally there is an overbite, but generally the bite is normal. Chin implant alone may be done, or the surgery may be performed in conjunction with a nose reconstruction.

A variety of implants have been advocated including bone from the patient's iliac crest (hip) and cartilage from the rib cage or the nose (harvested during a nose reconstruction). Additional tissue has been obtained from flaps or dermal fat grafts from the buttocks.

In recent years, silastic implants have gained in popularity. These are available in the form of preformed, gel-containing silastic bags or solid-block silastic contoured at the time of surgery. Acrylic implants also can be used. Injectable silicone is not an acceptable material at this time.

Time and Place: Mentoplasty can be an office or in-hospital procedure, and can be done under local or general anesthesia. The operation takes about three-quarters of an hour.

Preparation: Your face will be washed with an antiseptic solution and your mouth rinsed several times with an antiseptic mouthwash.

Procedure: An incision is placed either within the mouth (in front of the gums) or in the area below the chin. The implant is put into its pocket, and the site sutured. Restrictive dressings are applied to prevent shifting of the implants. Dressings are removed in three to four days.

Complications: Infection is always a potential threat with any non-living prosthesis used in chin augmentation. Wherever the incision is placed to accomplish the augmentation (intraorally or externally), malpositioning of the prosthesis is a possibility.

Cost: Ranges from $350–$1,000.

THE
BODY

The Body Silhouette

Purpose: To recontour the arms, legs, thighs, abdomen, or breasts in an aesthetically pleasing fashion.

Overview: Today's fashionable silhouette is tall and thin with small or moderate-sized breasts. Some of these characteristics must be engineered genetically; they fall outside the realm of the aesthetic surgeon. Others can be achieved to a reasonable extent by a regimen of proper diet and exercise. Good medical management is needed, as is much encouragement. Following successful dieting, however, many women are left with painfully visible stigmata of their recent shift in weight: the pendulous abdomen, sagging upper arms, sagging breasts, or full thighs and buttocks. To a great extent, these are correctable. One must emphasize, however, that while the contour can be improved, the resultant scars at the surgical sites will be visible on the body.

Besides dieters, a group that may wish to avail themselves of corrective abdominal surgery, are women with deformity of the abdomen following childbirth. (Naturally, we discourage women who have yet to complete their families from having this surgery.) Potential candidates for this procedure suffer such deformities as stretch marks of an extensive nature (striae); laxity of the skin and subcutaneous tissue; and separation of the abdominal musculature, sometimes leading to herniation of abdominal contents (diastasis recti).

Also, some women experience loss of skin tone and elasticity as part of the normal aging process. For these patients, an abdominal lipectomy, breast lift, or correction of sagging upper arms may be beneficial.

Here are detailed descriptions of the procedures for *abdominal lipectomy*. Corrective surgery for other areas of the body silhouette is outlined in the remaining section of this part of the book.

Abdominal Lipectomy

Time and Place: This surgery is almost always performed in a hospital. Hospitalization may last ten to fourteen days.

Preparation: You must eliminate excess fat by sensible dieting under medical supervision. After you achieve a reasonable weight, and are able to remain at that weight for at least six months, you can be scheduled for surgery.

On the night before surgery, you will be asked to shower, using an antiseptic solution such as Betadine® or Phisohex®. The pubic hairs will then be shaved. Your blood will be typed and cross-matched for possible transfusion; blood loss during this surgery can be considerable. Auto-transfusion, in which your own blood is taken beforehand and stored, is a technique that is gaining in popularity and has the advantage of minimizing the risk of transfusion reaction and hepatitis.

Procedure: There are two general categories of abdominal lipectomy patients. For the first, the patient with a huge abdominal apron that has developed as a result of extreme weight reduction, the goal is to reduce the volume of the abdomen. Scar placement is not given primary consideration, because this patient is unlikely to be interested in wearing bikini swimsuits or highly contoured clothing. A "belt lipectomy" is a suitable approach here.

A simple incision extending across the abdomen, possibly to the back at the level of the umbilicus, is made. The skin and fat extending above to the rib cage and below to the pubis are raised, and, by traction, the excess is removed. Any separation or herniation of the abdominal musculature is repaired, and the umbilicus is repositioned in its correct location. This procedure may entail considerable blood loss, and transfusions may be needed. In addition, drains placed beneath the flaps to prevent the collection of serum or blood may serve as a potential focus for infection. There are several modifications of this procedure. The choice is based on the surgeon's preference and is generally tailored to suit the individual patient.

A second category of abdominal lipectomy patients includes those with stretch marks, separation (diastasis) of musculature, or unacceptable scars from prior abdominal surgery. With these women, more care may be taken with the placement of the scar, particularly if the patient is eager to wear body-revealing clothing.

The incision is placed one-half to two centimeters below the pubic hairline, extending into the groin and then to the hip. A flap is raised to the ribcage above, and excess tissue is removed. The umbilicus is repositioned in its correct location. A small circular scar will extend around the umbilicus; the scar tends to fade with time. Stretch marks below the pubis and umbilicus will be removed; those above these areas will remain but will be less noticeable.

The wounds are closed in layers, using absorbable suture material in the depth and subcuticular closure supplemented by steri-tapes on the surface. This proce-

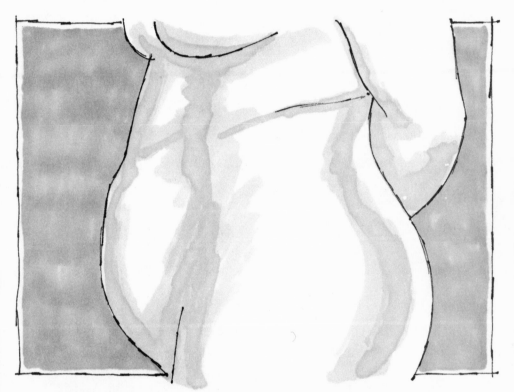

Abdominal Lipectomy—pre-op

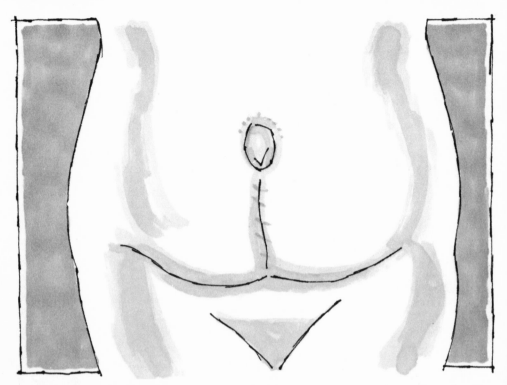

Abdominal Lipectomy—post-op, front view

dure prevents the development of track marks. Drains are placed and brought out through the most lateral portion of the wound. The patient is placed in a flexed position and kept in bed for several days to prevent undue stretching of the wound or potential wound separation.

Once allowed out of bed, the patient must wear a girdle to lend extra support and prevent wound separation. Drains are usually removed within forty-eight hours, after which the wound is redressed. The subcuticular sutures remain for at least two weeks, and the skin steri-tapes are kept in place as long as they remain adherent.

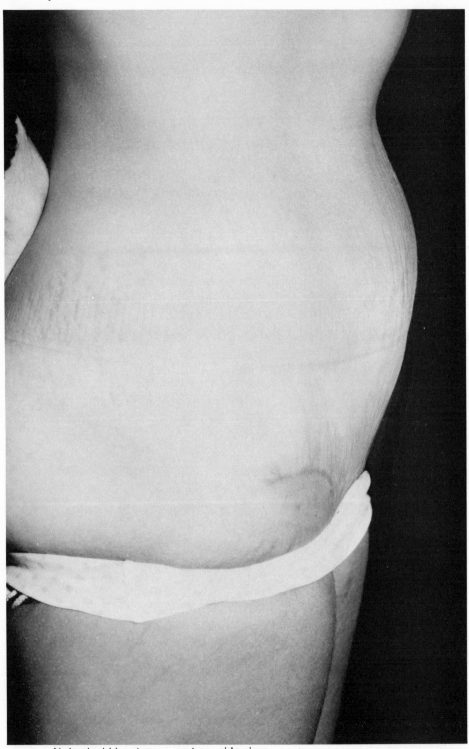

Abdominal Lipectomy—post-op, side view

Pain and Discomfort: A minimal amount of pain is associated with the procedure. Of more concern than pain to most patients is the inconvenience of being in a flexed position and having to remain in bed for several days.

Complications: Potential problems associated with this surgery are skin slough secondary to infected hematomas. Most often, conservative management results in a satisfactory outcome. Infection and hematomas (collections of blood) fortunately are infrequent. Fat necrosis is a potential hazard, but this is more of a risk in the extremely obese patient undergoing lipectomy. Blood loss can be considerable, and adequate replacement is a necessity.

Recurrence of the initial problem is usually not seen unless the patient fails to heed advice. For example, if you underwent surgery to remove stretch marks, a new pregnancy would certainly precipitate all the causes for the original operation.

Aftereffects: None except for scarring, which is unavoidable. You must indulge in only moderate activity for several weeks after surgery.

Cost: This procedure can cost $1,800–$3,500, depending on where you live and which surgeon you choose.

THE
BREASTS

Enlargement of the Breasts (Mammoplasty)

Purpose: To enlarge the breasts by placement of artificial implants.

Overview: This operation was designed to correct such conditions as underdevelopment (hypoplasia) and reduction of breast substance following childbirth or extreme weight loss. In selected patients, it may be used to correct the cosmetic deformity following mastectomy.

The implant, or prosthesis, is a silastic bag containing a polysiloxane gel. This is a slow-flowing gel that has a consistency much like that of the normal breast. After the placement of the implant, the body generally forms a fibrous capsule around the prosthesis, which reduces implant shifting and protects the prosthesis from injury. An implant may be ruptured by a penetrating puncture wound, however, or by a high-velocity impact injury. Fortunately, this is a rare event. There is no evidence at this time that the silastic bag or its contents are in any way cancer-producing.

Breast implants come in various shapes, such as teardrop, round, or oval. This is not an important considera-

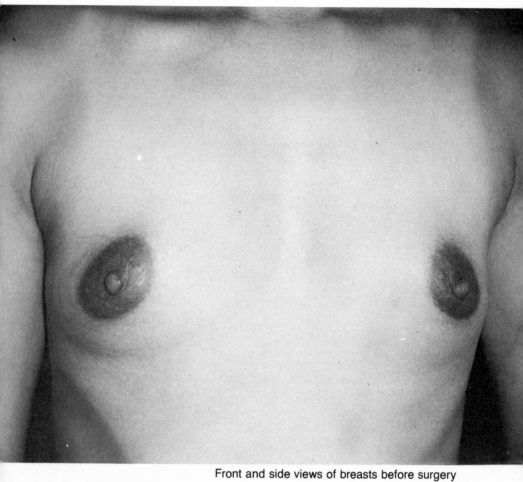

Front and side views of breasts before surgery

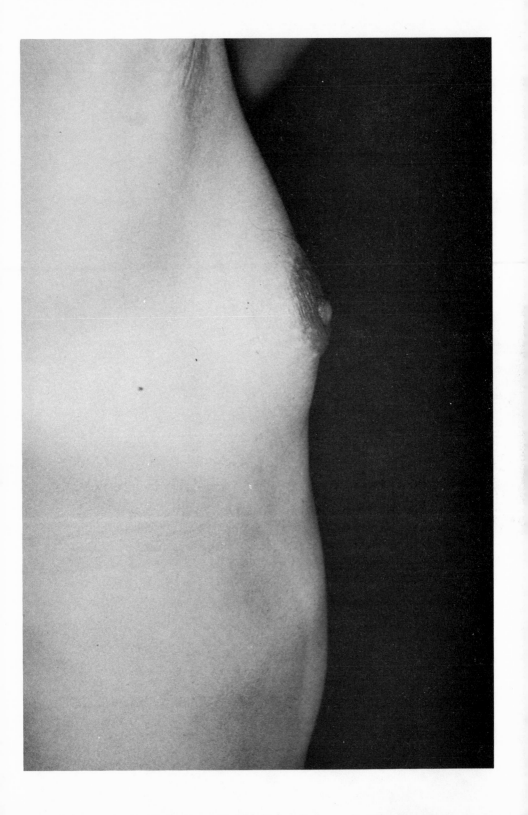

tion, because, after placement, the effects of gravity on the gel result in all implants looking rather similar. Size *is* an important consideration. Patients often request an unsuitably large implant, one that would create an artificial and disproportionate appearance. In this regard, it might be best to consider the brassiere size you desire. A cup size of B or C is a reasonable goal and can usually be achieved with an implant containing 190 cc of gel. Implants are available in volumes ranging from 165 to 450 cc. The latter implant, however, would probably produce a breast requiring a double-D cup.

Time and Place: The procedure generally takes about one and one-half hours to perform. It may be done in a hospital or in the surgeon's office, using general or local anesthesia. If you are hospitalized, prepare for a stay of three to five days.

Preparation: You will be asked to shower with an antiseptic solution. Preoperative sedation will be administered to alleviate enxiety.

Procedure: The patient is positioned on the table with her head elevated about 30 degrees and her hands fixed over her abdomen. This positioning aids in placing the prosthesis in a symmetrical and natural position. An incision three to five centimeters long is made approximately five centimeters beneath and just lateral to the nipple. (This incision ultimately falls into the crease created by the lower border of the breast.) A pocket is created through the incision, and this holds the prosthesis. It will lie in front of the chest wall muscle, but beneath any existing breast tissue. It is important to note this fact. Because the patient's own breast tissue lies over the prosthesis, the nipple maintains its connection to the ductal system of the breast and allows for nursing.

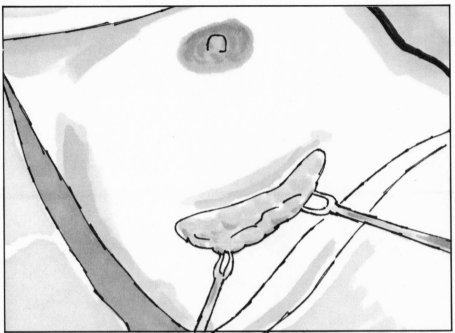

A pocket is cut into the tissue underneath the breast.

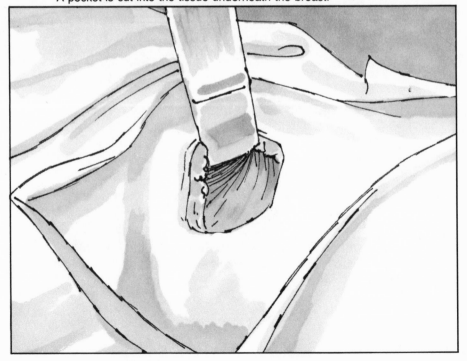

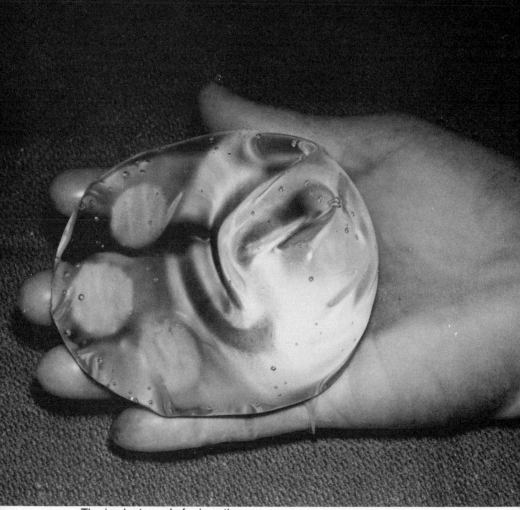

The implant, ready for insertion.

Surgical drains are generally not necessary except in cases with difficult dissection that might lead to excessive collections of blood (hematomas). If drains are placed, they are generally removed in twenty-four to forty-eight hours.

There are several alternate approaches with respect to placement of the incision. It may be placed within the nipple, in the armpit, or from an abdominal approach in conjunction with a panniculectomy in the abdomen. Your surgeon will discuss his choice with you prior to surgery.

Aftereffects: There is diminished sensation in the nipples as a result of stretching nerve endings over the implant. Generally, recovery of normal sensation occurs within a year following surgery. Some surgeons limit extreme stretching and the lifting of heavy objects for approximately six weeks, but others place no limitations on these activities. A jobst, Fredericks, or long-line support bra that buttons in front will provide added support. As stated, augmentation mammoplasty should not interfere with the ability to nurse.

After the implant is properly positioned, the tissue pocket is closed.

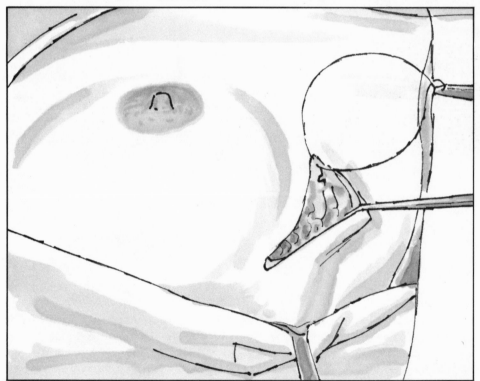

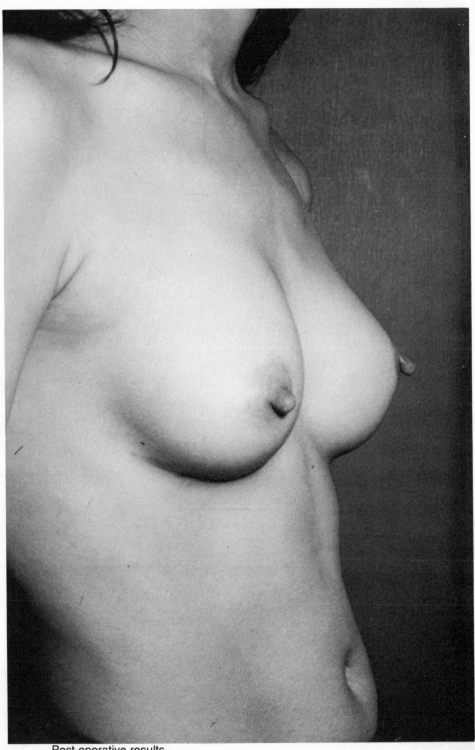

Post-operative results

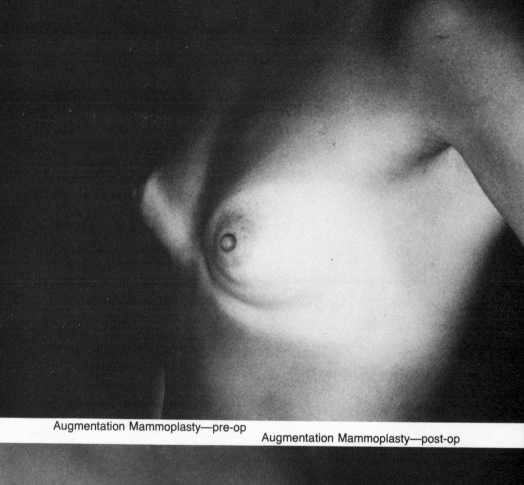

Augmentation Mammoplasty—pre-op   Augmentation Mammoplasty—post-op

Complications: A collection of blood (hematoma) may form beneath the skin. If this is small, it probably does not require any treatment. But if the collection is large and is causing you pain, drainage is necessary to relieve the pain and remove the blood, which can provide a suitable culture media for bacteria and lead to infection. Should you develop an infection, additional drainage and antibiotic therapy would be instituted.

Two possible complications may occur later. The first, excessive firmness of the breasts, results from a high degree of scarring (fibrous capsule formation). Some scar formation is expected and in fact desired. But hematomas and infections tend to stimulate too much scarring. The second late complication, extrusion of the implant, is very rare and obviously requires attention.

Cost: This ranges from $1,000–$3,000. Implants cost about $200 and are generally ordered by the physician.

Reduction of the Breasts
(Mammoplasty)

Purpose: To reduce large and unwieldy breasts to a more normal size and contour.

Overview: Various techniques involving excision of breast tissue are available for reducing breast size. Women seeking this type of surgery often complain of breast, back, and lower neck pain. Hypertrophic breasts may, in fact, be associated with arthritic changes of the cervical spine. This condition should be investigated before considering a mammoplasty. Another frequent complaint is that of grooving the shoulders secondary to pressure from brassiere straps. In addition, there may be considerable irritation beneath pendulous breasts, which is aggravated in the summer months by excessive perspiration. In rare instances, ulnar nerve injury leading to impairment of hand function is seen. Aside from any physical disabilities, considerable mental anguish can be associated with oversized breasts. Embarrassment resulting from this overdevelopment may prompt a woman to shun social contacts.

Aesthetic considerations dictate the size of the breast wanted after reduction. A generally acceptable goal is to achieve a volume of 250–300 cc, which translates to a C-cup brassiere size. An open and frank discussion with your surgeon regarding breast size should take place before surgery.

Preoperative evaluation should include an adequate physical examination of the breasts along with mammography or thermography. If there is any evidence of a breast mass of any significance, a biopsy is indicated, and this can be carried out at the time of the surgery. Should the biopsy prove malignant, appropriate treatment must be carried out. Obviously, reduction of the breast under these circumstances is not acceptable.

Endocrine gland malfunction should be considered during preoperative evaluation as well as other either metabolic or drug-induced causes for breast enlargement. In the drug category are medications such as Reserpine® and the oral contraceptives. Pregnancy can also cause considerable breast enlargement. Overweight women should be encouraged to lose weight and maintain the lower weight for several months before breast-reduction surgery is considered. And it is best to avoid surgery just prior to a menstrual period because of premenstrual breast enlargement.

The ideal age for carrying out this procedure is sixteen to twenty years old, but it has been done successfully in older women. Favorable healing takes place at this time and the social and physiologic benefits are optimal.

Reconstruction of the breast fulfills physiological as well as aesthetic needs. Women who undergo this surgery may experience improved posture and breathing and less physical discomfort generally. Unfortunately, because of manipulation of the position of the nipple, the ability to nurse is often lost.

Time and Place: This procedure is usually performed in a hospital under general anesthesia. The surgery takes three to four hours to complete . Hospital stay can be from three to five days.

Preparation: On the evening prior to the surgery, or on the morning of the operation, the surgeon will make markings on your breasts that will guide him during the procedure. These markings are arrived at after careful preoperative evaluation of breast size and contour. Photographs generally aid in this planning.

In an attempt to avoid the risks associated with blood transfusions (e.g., hepatitis, transfusion reactions), many physicians have been encouraging the use of auto-transfusions. If this is done in your case, your blood will be removed on several occasions over a few weeks prior to surgery and stored for you at the hospital. Your body will have replenished much of the withdrawn blood by the time of surgery, and you will have your own blood available for transfusion should you need it. If you object to transfusions (auto or donor) on a religious basis, you may not be a suitable candidate for this surgery, as blood loss can be considerable.

On the day of the surgery, you will shower with an antiseptic solution. Preoperative sedation will then be administered.

Procedure: *The Strombeck-Wise Technique.* There are many techniques described for reduction mammoplasty and each has its advocates. Your surgeon will choose what he deems best for you. The technique described here is a standard procedure that serves as a basis for other surgical approaches and is presented only as an example. A pattern much like one for a garment is used as a guide to the excision of the excess breast tissue and relocation of the nipple. Using the standard pattern along with appropriate measurements, the new nipple site is located.

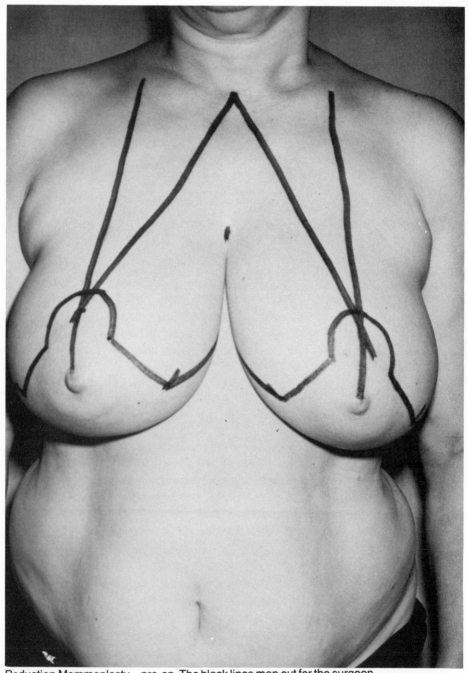

Reduction Mammoplasty—pre-op. The black lines map out for the surgeon how the breasts are to be re-shaped.

The limbs of the breast flaps are determined. A split-thickness skin graft is removed to create a dermal pedicle, which will be the source of blood supply to the newly placed nipple. This new nipple site is prepared by excising a small amount of breast tissue. Resection of excess breast tissue is then carried out following the previously outlined pattern. The tissue removed from each breast is weighed in order to help achieve maximum symmetry of the two breasts. The nipple is then moved into its new location and sutured into place. Further suturing of the breast is carried out, producing the desired conical shape. Drains are placed on the outer aspect of the lower suture line. The final skin closure results in an inverted "T"-shaped scar. Dressings are applied to provide compression and support for the breasts. The dressings remain in place for several days. Drains are usually removed after forty-eight hours. A support bra is often recommended after the initial dressing change.

Pain and Discomfort: You will experience mild to moderate pain; excessive pain suggests the development of a complication. Most pain will respond to mild analgesics and will subside in about twenty-four hours.

Complications: The overall complication rate falls below 10 percent and, fortunately, the more severe complications are considerably less frequent. Early problems may include discoloration of the nipple and areolar area, which may reflect a localized collection of blood with resultant infection, or stitch abscesses. You may also see small wound separations, small areas of skin necrosis, and inclusion cysts along the suture line. More serious complications include partial or complete loss of the nipple, loss of skin, fat necrosis, and, rarely, loss of portions of breast tissue.

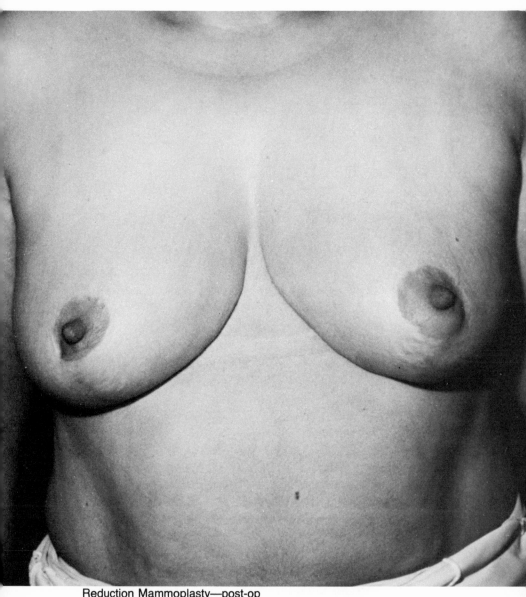

Reduction Mammoplasty—post-op

Long-term complications may include asymmetry of the breasts, which can result from one or more of the above problems. Spreading of scars, nipple retraction, malposition of the areola and nipple, inability to nurse, and decreased breast sensation of a temporary or permanent nature are possible.

Cost: The procedure costs $1,800–$4,500.

Correction of Drooping Breasts (Maxstopexy)

Purpose: To correct ptosis (drooping breasts).

Overview: Ptosis is defined as the drooping of the breast so that the nipple lies beneath the line representing the inframammary fold (i.e., on the underside of the breast). Several factors are known to contribute to the development of drooping breasts, the most common being postpartum hypoplasia, which is an actual loss of breast volume following childbirth. A second factor is the effect of gravity on the supporting tissues of the breast. To understand this, it may help to view the breast as an envelope containing tissue. Overstretching this envelope can result in a drooping, pancake-like appearance to the breast.

Women who wish this surgery may have very small ptotic breasts or very large ptotic breasts. In the former case, augmentation mammoplasty plus resuspension of the breasts is indicated. In the latter, breast reduction (excision of excess breast tissue) along with resuspension can be performed. In all these procedures, the breast is resuspended and the nipple surgically relocated.

Women whose breast size is adequate may be consid-

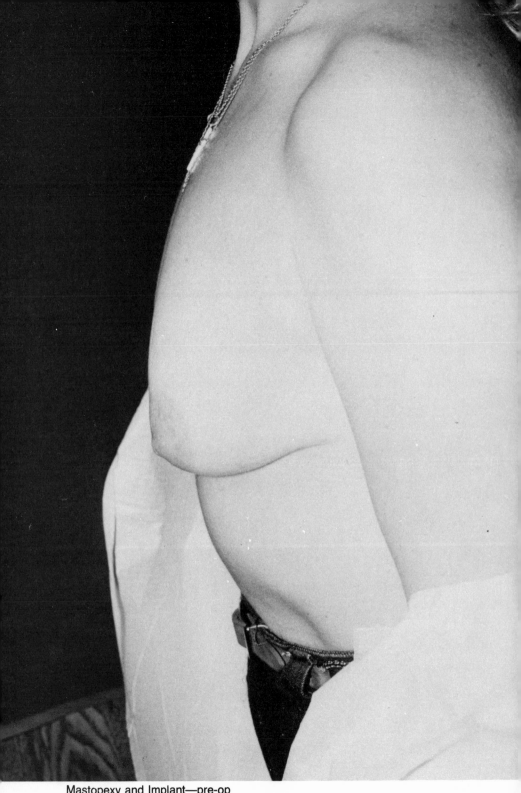

Mastopexy and Implant—pre-op

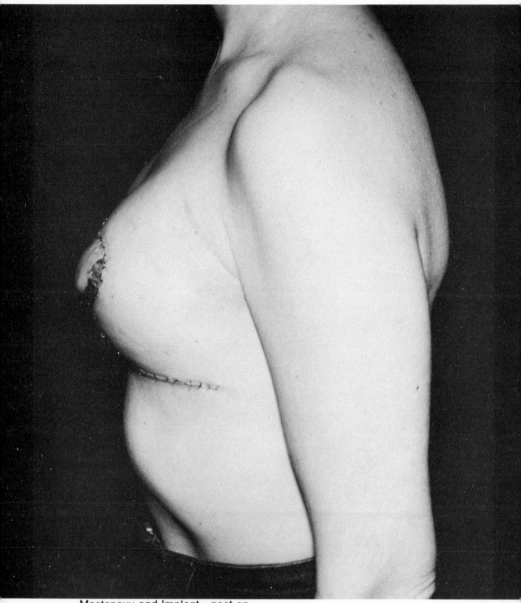

Mastopexy and Implant—post-op

ering a mastopexy because the nipples fall on the underside of the breasts or point downward. Corrective surgery of this type can be performed at any age, but obviously should be avoided soon after pregnancy, when swelling is still considerable. Generally, women in their late thirties and early forties seek this surgery. A woman who has undergone weight reduction should put off this surgery until her weight has stabilized and the lower weight has been maintained for several months.

Women with mild asymmetry of the breasts may also be helped by this procedure.

Time and Place: In simple cases, this surgery can be performed in an outpatient facility under local anesthesia. More commonly, the surgery is done in a hospital under general anesthesia. The operation takes about two hours, but if reduction or augmentation is also performed, the procedure takes considerably longer. A hospital stay of three to five days is usual.

Preparation: You will be asked to shower with an antiseptic solution. Preoperative sedation will be administered to alleviate anxiety.

Procedure: In cases of simple ptosis, markings are made preoperatively on the breasts in order to determine the new position of the nipples. At surgery, the planned site for the nipples are denuded of superficial layers of skin. The nipples are repositioned and sutured in place. The breast tissue is then tightened with sutures, and a small amount of excess breast and skin tissue may be trimmed inferiorly. A dressing is applied and is left in place for two to three weeks. Drains are generally not necessary.

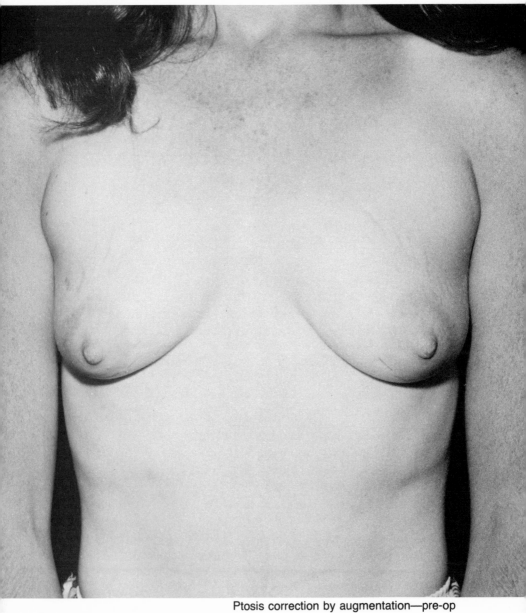

Ptosis correction by augmentation—pre-op

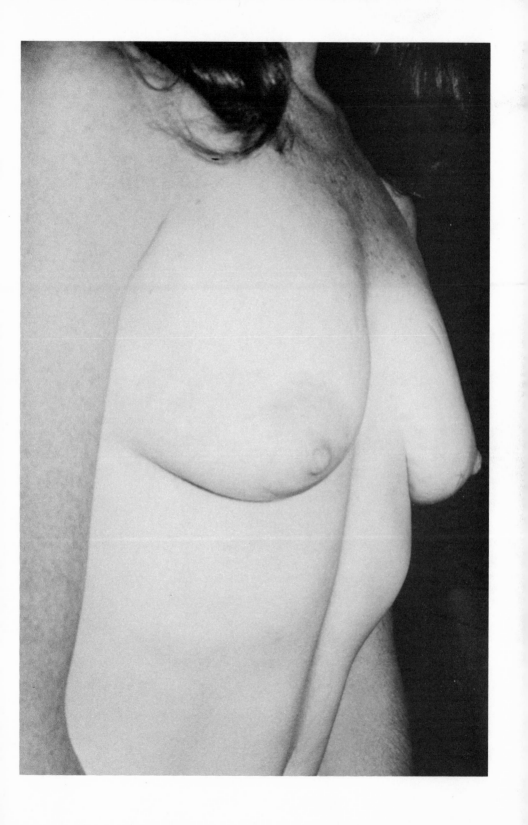

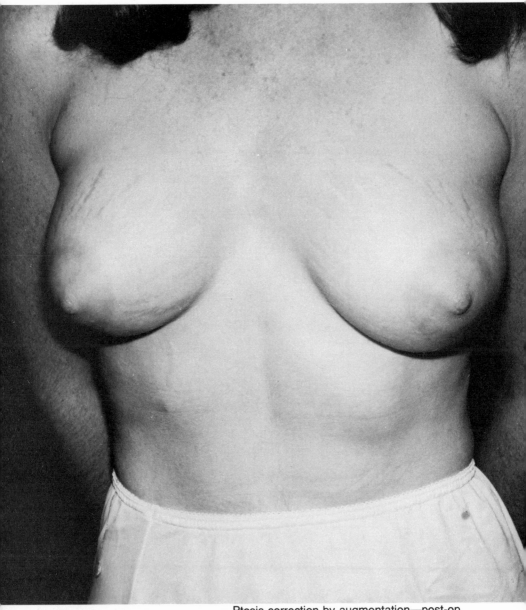

Ptosis correction by augmentation—post-op

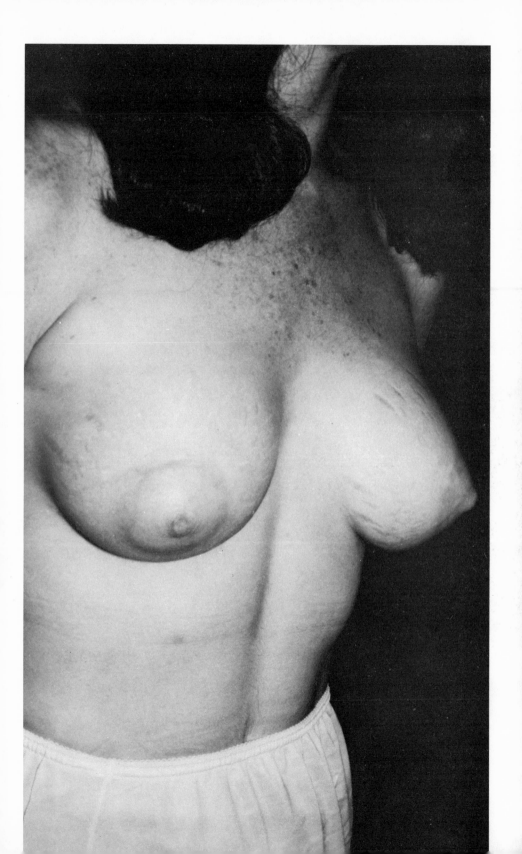

Complications: Surgical scars on the breast may become more visible on stretching, especially if you gain weight or become pregnant. A serious but uncommon complication is necrosis with loss of the nipple.

Pain and Discomfort: Expect some pain, but prolonged pain may indicate a complication such as hematoma (collection of blood under the skin), infection, or wound separation. Fortunately, all are uncommon.

Cost: The procedure costs $1,500–$4,000.

Breast Reconstruction After Mastectomy

Purpose: To re-create the breast in women who have undergone mastectomy for cancer.

Overview: The loss of a breast can lead to significant psychological difficulties. Coupled with the fear associated with having cancer, a woman may experience a sense of loss of femininity and diminished self-image. Over the years, many procedures have been devised in an attempt to reconstruct the lost breast. Success has been variable and the procedures are often lengthy and fraught with complications. Questions have been raised regarding the appropriate time interval between mastectomy and reconstruction, and the propriety of breast reconstruction after mastectomy. These questions are based on the knowledge that the average time the patient will remain free of disease is 43 months, and that reconstruction performed before this time interval may obscure the recognition of renewed disease. However, with the perfection of diagnostic techniques and the overwhelming desire of the patients to be "whole again" the pendulum is swinging in favor of early reconstruction.

The consensus now favors breast reconstruction, and some surgeons even advocate performing it immediately following the mastectomy. In attempting to establish criteria for suitable candidates for surgery, we have found the following guidelines useful:

1. There should be no evidence of persistence of disease at the site of mastectomy, nor should there be any clinical or laboratory evidence of metastatic disease.

2. The skin and underlying tissue at the mastectomy site should be in suitable condition to withstand surgical manipulation. For example, if radiation therapy has been administered, the resultant radiation dermatitis will complicate reconstructive efforts. The presence of a skin graft also will necessitate a more complicated surgical technique.

3. The opposite breast should be free of disease.

4. A prospective patient should fully understand the limitations and potential complications of any reconstructive procedure. Psychological screening may be helpful here to determine if the woman is a suitable candidate for surgery.

Timing of Reconstruction: Reconstruction can be performed at any time from two days to three years after a mastectomy. Recurrence of disease is most likely within five years; the average is forty-three months. Thus it is difficult to dictate guidelines for the ideal time for reconstruction. The scheduling must be flexible and take into account the following:

- General health of the patient
- Age of the patient
- Type of tumor (which may aid in predicting its behavior)
- Mental well-being of the patient
- Marital status of the patient

• Condition of the chest-wall tissues

The ideal candidate for early reconstruction is a young woman whose initial lesion was small, who has no evidence of a persistent disease, and who is motivated to have the reconstructive surgery.

Preparation: You will be asked to shower with an antiseptic solution. Preoperative sedation will be administered to alleviate anxiety.

Procedure: In women on whom a simple mastectomy or modified radical mastectomy has been performed, and where the major muscle group is still intact, a prosthesis (implant) may be placed beneath the skin or beneath the muscle. An incision is made and the skin and muscle raised so that an appropriately sized prothesis may be slipped into the pocket. The incision site should then fall into the inframammary fold.

The preceding description applies to a relatively uncomplicated radical mastectomy operative site. In the event that the guidelines for uncomplicated reconstruction are not met, other techniques are now available to effect reconstruction. These include the latissimus dorsi flap (a musculocutaneous flap) i.e. tissue consisting of skin and muscle as a single unit that can be transferred with its own intact blood supply to reconstruct the entire breast that has been removed. The donor site for this flap is on the lateral part of the back. This is a highly successful flap and solves many of the problems found where there was adequate skin coverage for reconstruction. This procedure is usually one stage with a brief second stage for nipple grafting.

The complications described below are much reduced if the flap technique is used.

There are other procedures available in cases where there are the following problems: radiation damage, deficiency of skin secondary to the type of surgical procedure performed (radical mastectomy with skin graft), or changes secondary to fibrosis and scarring as a result of adjunctive chemotherapy. These may include procedures such as the musculocutaeous flap (for example, the latissimus dorsi flap). Other flaps also used for this defect are the thoraco abdominal flap or the medially based abdominal flap. (A flap is full thickness tissue that is moved from one side of the body to another creating a defect from the site from which it is taken to correct a problem elsewhere.)

Complications: These are similar to the complications following augmentation mammoplasty: collections of blood (hematomas), infection, skin loss, and potential extrusion of the prosthesis. A late complication is the formation of a scar around the implant, which can lead to a globular appearance.

The most significant complication is that of disease recurrence. That the disease recurs is not related to the presence of the implant, but the prosthesis may make early detection more difficult. Because of this, mammography is a useful follow-up tool for women who have undergone breast reconstruction.

Cost: The procedure costs $2500–$6000.

Correction of
Male Breast Enlargement
(Gynecomastia)

Purpose: To correct any benign enlargement of the male breast.

Overview: Enlargement of breast tissue in males may be associated with considerable anxiety and psychological difficulties. This is particularly true in adolescent and young adult males. A fear of ridicule may prompt males with this condition to avoid any activity that necessitates baring the chest.

The underlying causes of male breast enlargement are varied. The most common cause is puberty with its hormonal changes. All patients should be evaluated appropriately prior to surgery, however.

Corrective procedures vary with the degree of deformity. They are classified according to the degree of skin excess associated with the enlargement of breast tissue.

Time and Place: Surgery is performed in the hospital under general anesthesia. Operating time is two to three hours if both breasts require correction.

Preparation: The surgical site is shaved on the evening prior to surgery, and the patient is instructed to shower with an antiseptic solution.

Procedure: An incision made on the edge of the nipple is extended in a half-moon shape along the perimeter of the nipple. This skin is raised from the underlying breast, and, by careful dissection, prominent tissue is removed. The wound is closed and a compression dressing applied. With this technique, it is possible to remove a considerable amount of tissue through a rather small incision.

In patients with skin excess, an elliptical excision of the excess skin is carried out along with dissection of breast tissue. The nipple must then be reimplanted.

If the procedure is extensive, drains are sometimes used to prevent blood accumulation. Generally, a compression dressing is sufficient.

Aftereffects and Complications: Hematoma formation (bleeding beneath the skin) is always a risk when the dissection is extensive, and can lead to infection and delayed healing. Late complications include persistence of skin excess; inverted, folded, or retroverted nipples; depression concavity of the nipples; and, occasionally, residual breast enlargement. Keloids, enlarged scars that extend beyond the incision site, sometimes form.

Cost: This procedure costs $850–$1,500.

THE LIMBS

Upper Arm Reconstruction (Dermolipectomy)

Purpose: To remove sagging skin and fat on the gravity-dependent area of the upper arm.

Overview: Persons who seek dermolipectomy of the upper arms often have lost considerable weight, which has resulted in severe sagging of the skin on the arms. This sagging may, in fact, extend onto the chest wall. Other candidates for this surgery have inherited the characteristic of excessive fat on the upper arms. Whatever the reason, the condition can cause considerable embarrassment when the person is wearing a swimsuit or arm-revealing apparel. Because corrective surgery results in scarring, anyone contemplating this surgery must weigh the potential benefits carefully. Those with a minimal degree of deformity are advised against undergoing surgery.

Time and Place: This is an in-hospital procedure performed under general anesthesia. Operating time is approximately two and one-half hours. Hospital stay is generally three to five days.

Preparation: You will be asked to shower with an antiseptic solution. Preoperative sedation will be administered.

Procedure: On the evening prior to surgery, markings are made with the patient in an upright position with the arms extended to the sides and perpendicular to the body. At the time of surgery, these markings serve as a road map to guide the surgeon's incisions. The excess tissue is removed and tightened from the elbow to the underarm. The wound margins are sutured beneath the skin and taped together at the surface. Drains are generally not required. A bulky compression dressing is applied.

Aftereffects: Postoperatively, two to three days of immobilization are recommended. The patient is positioned with the arms away from the chest wall and elevated on pillows. Moving the wrists is recommended, however. Pain and swelling are generally minimal. Most patients are discharged with a light dressing; sutures (or tapes) are removed in about two weeks. Some surgeons tape the wound edges with steri-strips for two to three months postoperatively to reduce spreading of the scar.

Complications: There can be wound separation and loss of a portion of skin along the suture line. Irregularities in the contour of the arms can occur. Residual tissue is possible around the elbows or armpits; this is more apt to happen in severely obese patients. There are sometimes hypertrophic (thickened) scars. Permanent swelling of the extremity can result from lymphatic blockage.

Cost: The average price is $1,500–$4,000.

Correction of
Thigh and Buttock Deformity
(Dermolipectomy)

Purpose: To correct trochanteric lipodystrophy, commonly known as the "love handle" deformity.

Overview: This protrusion of the upper lateral thighs and buttocks results from an accumulation of fat and is also often associated with a depression in this region. For many persons with this condition, bulging thighs resulting from excess weight can be corrected by diet and exercise. For others, however, no amount of exercise or weight reduction will correct the deformity. This condition appears to be genetically determined.

Surgical candidates are advised to lose weight and maintain the lower weight level for a period of six months or longer. Of course, the weight loss must be accomplished in a sensible and controlled fashion to avoid metabolic problems that could compromise the surgery. It should be noted at this point that the weight reduction will make the protrusion of the thighs appear more prominent. But this is unavoidable and temporary. If you are unable to approach ideal weight, you are probably not a suitable candidate for this surgery.

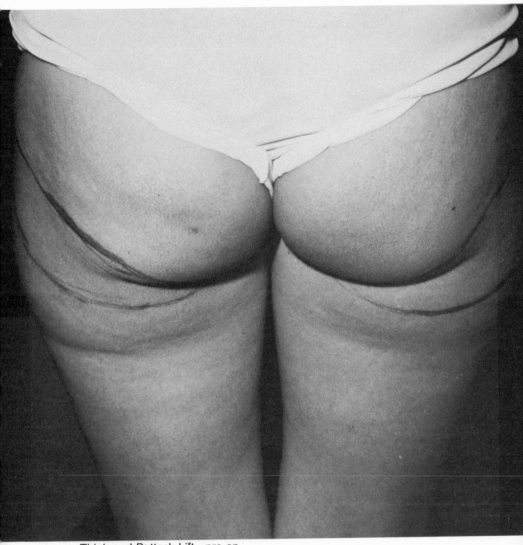

Thigh and Buttock Lift—pre-op

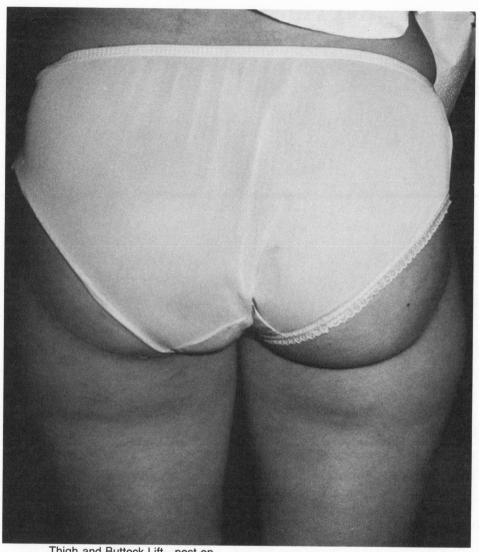

Thigh and Buttock Lift—post-op

Time and Place: This procedure is usually performed in a hospital under general anesthesia. Operating time is approximately two and one-half hours. Hospital stay can vary from three to seven days, and some patients are discharged two days after surgery.

Preparation: You will be bathed in an antiseptic solution. Any hair that will be in the line of excision will be removed. Preoperative markings of the lines of excision will be made on the evening prior to surgery with indelible ink or scratch marks. These markings should be made while you are standing because the deformity is most apparent in that position.

Procedure: With the patient lying face down, incisions are made from the gluteal fold (of the buttocks) out to the lateral thighs, in the area of the gluteal crease. A wedge of skin and subcutaneous tissue wide enough to encompass both fatty and depressed areas is removed. The wound edges are then brought together and sutured. These sutures remain in place for eight to fourteen days. (Some surgeons prefer to suture with wire beneath the skin and paper tape along the skin surface.)

Complications: Because of constant tension along the suture lines, spreading scars are common. If you gain weight or become pregnant, the deformity may recur. Occasionally, there is difficulty in achieving a harmonious curve on the thigh. This may be accentuated by the development of a depressed scar. Phlebitis, an inflammation of the veins, is the most serious complication, and is most apt to occur in the severely obese patient.

Cost: $1,500–$4,500.

Correction of Lax Skin on Thighs (Crural Meloplasty)

Purpose: To correct thin, lax skin on the thigh near the groin.

Overview: Sagging skin in the area of the groin occurs as tissues relax and aging progresses. Lax thigh skin is especially prominent on people who have undergone considerable weight loss. The resultant formation of pouching and bagging skin is unsightly and can lead to skin irritation caused by friction and perspiration.

Time and Place: This surgery can be performed in a hospital or in a well-equipped clinic. General anesthesia is usually administered. Operating-room time is about two and one-half hours.

Preparation: The groin area will be shaved on the evening prior to surgery. This will be followed by an antiseptic bath or shower.

Procedure: Incisions are made in the inner aspect of the upper thigh. These incisions extend along the groin crease halfway around the front and back of the thigh. A wedge of excess tissue is removed, and the skin is pulled taut and sutured beneath and on the surface of the skin. A simple modification may be performed if the tissue excess is confined to the inner thigh. In this situation, the incision is made in the groin crease, and about one centimeter of skin and underlying fat are removed. The excess fat is scooped out from this incision over the area of the maximum bulge. Sutures are placed, and a compression dressing, which must remain in place for about a month, is applied.

Aftereffects and Complications: Immediate problems can include hematoma formation (bleeding beneath the skin) and subsequent infection with secondary healing. Adequate drainage and antibiotics usually handle this problem. Long-term aftereffects can include stretching of the scar or scar migration inferiorly onto the visible area of the thigh.

Cost: This procedure costs $1,500–$4,000.

THE
HAIR

Hair Transplantation

Purpose: To resurface the scalp with hair following its loss from a variety of causes, most commonly that of male-pattern baldness.

Overview: Both men and women can benefit from this technique, which may also be useful in treating certain diseases affecting the hair or the scalp.

The principle of hair transplantation is based on the concept of "donor dominance." In male-pattern baldness, the hair loss always occurs in the central region of the scalp. Some less fortunate individuals also lose their hair along the border of the scalp, although generally not as extensively. In most cases, however, the border hair does not grow thinner. In hair transplantation, hairs taken from the border (donor site) with the aid of an instrument called a "punch" are moved to the hairless central region. These donor hairs will continue to behave as though they were still in their original site. That is, they will grow as they would have along the border of the scalp despite the fact that they have now been placed in a bald region. Male-pattern baldness is the most common complaint for

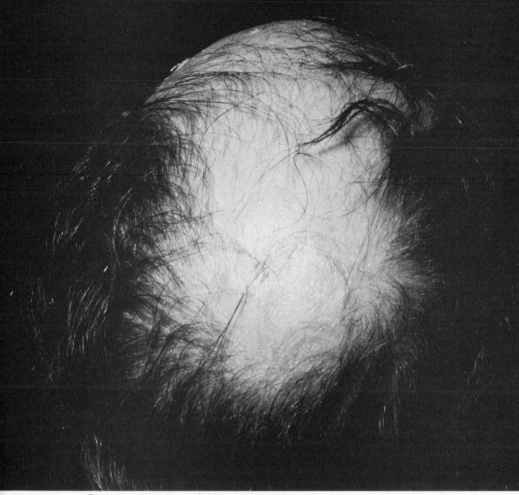

Pre-operative view prior to transplant.

which this technique is effective, but it also may be used on sites that become bald as a result of scars secondary to burns, surgery, or radiation therapy.

Recently, considerable notice has been given to techniques involving the movement of large flaps of hair-bearing scalp to bald areas. This procedure is carried out under a general anesthetic. Its advantage over the punch technique is that it achieves a more rapid correction. Nevertheless, the cosmetic effect may not be as pleasing as that achieved by the punch technique. Occasionally, a combination of flap and punch grafting may be the most satisfactory answer.

Preparation for Punch Graft Transplantation: A vigorous shampooing with an antiseptic solution such as Betadine® will be carried out by the patient on the evening prior to, and again on the morning of, surgery. This shampooing reduces the number of bacteria on the scalp and thus reduces the risk of infection.

Procedure: In the operating suite the scalp is washed with an antiseptic solution. The donor-site hairs are clipped short. This simplifies harvesting the donor grafts and makes it easier to determine the direction of hair growth so that the new hairs may be suitably oriented in the recipient (bald) site. After clipping, a local anesthetic is injected into both donor and recipient sites, rendering them free of pain during the procedure. The local anesthetic also contains epinephrine, which helps reduce bleeding. The donor grafts are then harvested with a round instrument (a punch), the head of which is generally 3–4 mm in size. The hairs and that portion of the scalp from which they grow are removed so as not to damage the growth center of the hair. This "donor plug" contains an average of ten growing hairs. The plug is trimmed of fat and floated in a petri dish containing sterile salt solution or placed on a moistened gauze until the recipient site is ready to receive it. The number of plugs transplanted at any session is generally decided on prior to the procedure and ranges from thirty to seventy. These donor sites may be sutured or may be left to close by shrinkage, depending upon the surgeon's preference.

The recipient site (the bald area) is readied by removing a series of punches measuring 3.5 mm in a number equal to that of the donor plugs. The donor plugs are placed into the recipient sites, taking care to orient them to grow in a direction that will appear natural. The recipient site is dressed with a bulky pressure dressing, which may be removed by the patient in twenty-four hours. Generally,

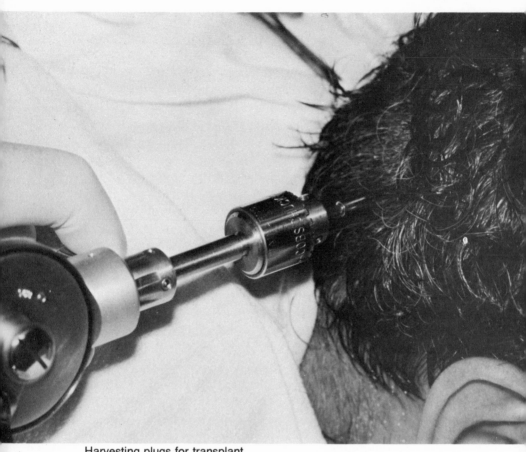
Harvesting plugs for transplant.

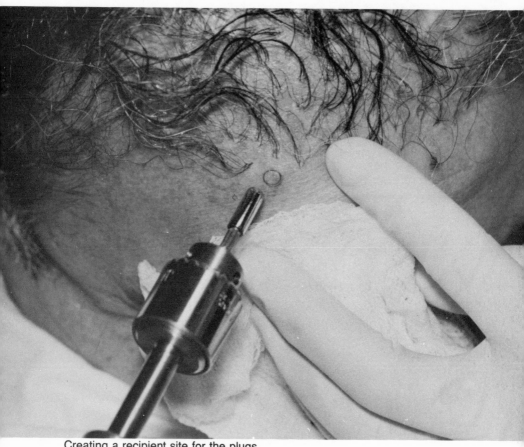

Creating a recipient site for the plugs.

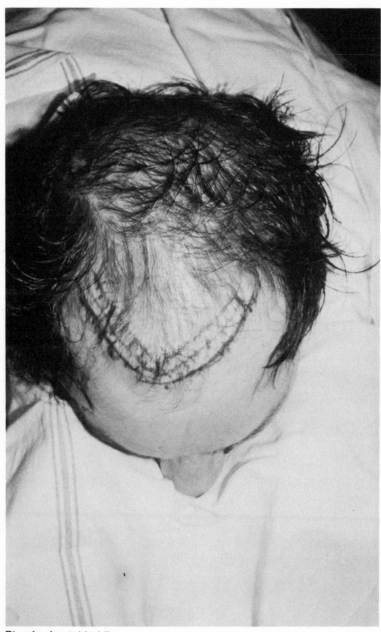

Plan for frontal hairline.

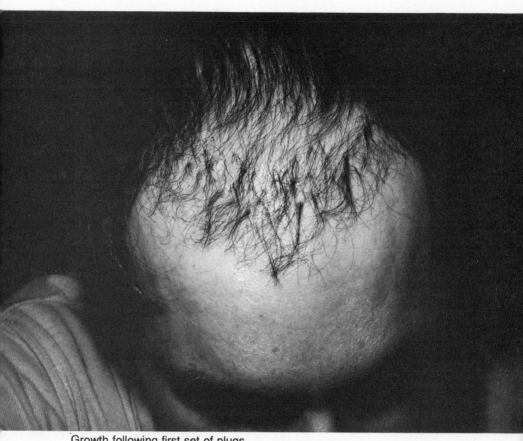

Growth following first set of plugs.

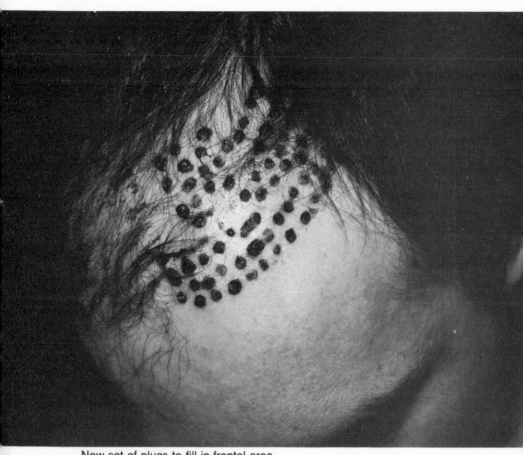

New set of plugs to fill in frontal area.

the hair can be washed about seven days after surgery. Vigorous exercise and bending must be avoided for one to two weeks after surgery.

Time and Place: This varies with the surgeon and of course with the number of plugs. A reasonable estimate would be forty-five minutes to one hour for sixty plugs. This procedure may be performed in your surgeon's office, in a clinic, or in the hospital.

Pain and Discomfort: Discomfort comes mainly from injections of the local anesthetic, which must be administered to all operative sites (donor and recipient). Anesthesia is generally achieved immediately; after that, the procedure should be painless. When the anesthesia wears off, throbbing pain may develop for about twenty-four hours but generally responds to mild oral analgesics.

Special Considerations: The most important criterion for success is that the donor-site hairs are of suitable density. The mere presence of a fringe of hair is not sufficient; plugs containing fewer than ten hairs or very thin hairs will not result in a sufficiently dense appearance on the recipient site. One can generally anticipate almost 100 percent survival of the plugs and approximately 95 percent of the hairs contained therein. Depending on the degree of baldness, the number of plugs transplanted may vary between 250 and 500. Surgery is generally carried out at intervals of six to eight weeks and thus can take a year or more to complete. This procedure requires patience and a stick-with-it attitude to achieve the desired result. In addition, the patient has to endure a period of hair loss on the newly transplanted site. This hair loss can begin immediately after transplant and last for several months before new hair growth begins.

Aftereffects and Complications: Bleeding, which may be controlled by direct pressure or suturing, is the most common problem. Patients with high blood pressure are the more likely candidates for this problem. The incidence of bleeding is reduced if exercise and bending are avoided. Actual loss of grafts is uncommon.

Cost: The cost per plug ranges from $15–$25.

THE
SKIN

Chemical Peel
(Chemoexfoliation)

Purpose: To reduce or eliminate fine wrinkling of the face, to treat superficial acne scarring, to correct pigmentary problems, or to reduce skin damage resulting from radiation.

Overview: The chemical peel is a technique that utilizes a phenol or a trichloracetic acid preparation to create a superficial burn on the upper layers of the skin. When these layers peel, the regrowing skin has a smoother appearance. The technique is effective in the treatment of fine vertical wrinkles around the mouth, crow's feet about the eyes, fine mosaic lines of the cheeks, and frown lines between the eyebrows. Not every individual can utilize this technique advantageously. The ideal patient is fair-complexioned and thin-skinned, with skin that has had a limited exposure to the outdoors. After treatment, delicate, thin skin yields a smooth, textured, and uniformly pigmented appearance. Darker-complexioned persons with a thick and oily skin would probably be poor candidates for a peel, particularly if they have a history of prolonged exposure to the sun. Because the peel tends to alter the degree of pigmentation of the skin, lines of demarcation between treated and untreated areas may be obvious on darker skin.

Chemical peel does not correct the sagging or laxity associated with aging, so it cannot be considered in place of a face lift. Rather, it should be used as an adjunct to the face lift, to effect a more favorable cosmetic result. Generally, the peel is most beneficial in treating wrinkles around the mouth; it is best performed about three weeks after a face lift.

Time and Place: The procedure can be performed in a well-equipped clinic or a hospital. In-hospital, it is generally done in the patient's room. The procedure takes about an hour. A hospital stay may last a week to ten days.

Preparation: Because you must be fully relaxed, sedation will be given about forty-five minutes prior to surgery. A solvent such as ether will be used to cleanse your skin of its natural oils.

The chemical peel to be applied consists of phenol, Croton oil, and septisol (an antiseptic solution). Each batch is freshly made up at the time of application. Trichloroacetic acid, in a 50-percent strength, is sometimes used instead of phenol. When this is used, the application differs considerably from the phenol procedure.

Phenol Procedure: The phenol solution is applied with a cotton-tipped applicator, generally beginning with the forehead and proceeding to the remainder of the face up to the area beneath the jaw. Fine wrinkles about the mouth are the particular target of the chemical peel. After the application is completed, waterproof tape is applied in two layers and must remain in place for forty-eight hours. During that time, most patients experience burning sensations of a considerable degree.

Aftereffects: Speaking should be avoided. You will be placed on a liquid diet to avoid chewing. Your face will become progressively more swollen; your eyes may shut completely. After about twenty-four hours, the skin will begin to weep and you may experience a wet sensation.

Forty-eight hours after surgery the dressing will be removed. Your face will have the appearance of a second-degree burn with redness, swelling, and blistering. Thymol-iodide powder will be applied; this forms a golden brown crust. The powder will be applied several times over the next twenty-hour hours.

An ointment such as Bacitracin® or A & D ointment® will be applied to the crusts three times daily until they separate, which usually occurs within a week. In general, you must stay in the hospital until the crusts have separated.

Trichloroacetic Acid Procedure: Trichloroacetic acid is also applied with a cotton-tipped applicator. A frost develops immediately on applying the chemical. A burning sensation is noted by the patient. The acid is left in place for five minutes, after which it is neutralized by an application of benzalkonium chloride (Zephiran®). The treated site is then washed with saline, and Bacitracin® ointment is applied. The pain generally subsides following the applicaton of the ointment. No dressing is used.

Aftereffects: The surgical site will be treated three to four times daily with a saline spray, followed by the application of Bacitracin®. Healing will take place over the next ten to fourteen days.

Pain and Discomfort: There is a moderate degree of discomfort and pain, probably more with phenol than with trichloroacetic acid.

Complications: Complications can arise from delayed healing, itching, milia formation (keloid-scar microcysts), and abnormal pigmentation. Occasionally there is pustule formation, which can be treated with antibiotics, and a prolonged redness that can last up to sixteen weeks postoperatively. Hypertrophic scar tissue formation is rare. Pigmented lesions present on the face prior to the peel may be darkened by the procedure and may be misinterpreted as a malignant change.

Cost: Cost varies with the area or areas to be treated and may range between $500 and $1,500.

Dermabrasion

Purpose: To reduce scarring resulting from acne, chicken pox, smallpox, radiodermatitis, trauma, and tattoos.

Overview: Dermabrasion is a procedure that utilizes a high-speed mechanical abrader to remove the superficial outer layers of the skin. When the skin grows back, it fills in the defects that are the residue of the disorders that produced the scarring. The technique is most often used for the correction of acne scars. Most surgeons recommend that the procedure be considered only for patients who no longer have an active skin condition or disease or whose condition is controlled. There are surgeons, however, who feel that active acne is not a contraindication for dermabrasion and may, in fact, lead to a reduction in the activity of the skin problem.

The results of dermabrasion vary with the depth of the scars, the depth to which the dermabrasion is carried out, and the number of times the procedure is performed at a given site. Raised scars respond most favorably, flat or pitted scars are treated successfully to a lesser degree, and

deeply pitted scars may require multiple abrasions at six-
to eight-week intervals.

In addition to treating scars, dermabrasion has proved
beneficial in the treatment of face wrinkles, although
it is not recommended for wrinkling around the mouth.

Time and Place: This procedure can be done in the surgeon's office or in a hospital. It takes about an hour to
complete. If you are hospitalized, expect a two-day stay.

Preparation: If acne is active, antibiotic therapy will be
administered prior to and following surgery. Preoperative
sedation, commonly Demerol®, morphine, or Valium®,
will be administered intramuscularly.

Procedure: If the surgery is performed in the doctor's
office, ethyl chloride is the usual anesthesia. Sprayed on
the skin, this chemical freezes the skin for fifteen to thirty
seconds. The face is divided into zones, each zone approximately four inches square. During the seconds in
which the skin is anesthesized, dermabrasion is carried
out. Superficial layers of skin are removed, section by
section, until all sites that are to be treated are done. Dermabrasion is possible on cheeks, chin, forehead, and
nose; it is not a suitable procedure for scars on the neck.
Although there is little or no pain involved in dermabrasion, each freeze and thaw may cause some discomfort.

In the hospital, dermabrasion can be performed with
the aid of a general or local anesthetic. In this case, the
spray is not necessary.

Pain and Discomfort: In addition to the discomfort of the
freeze-and-thaw period, postoperative pain similar to that
of a second-degree burn can be expected for about
twenty-four to forty-eight hours. Analgesics will generally relieve the pain.

Aftereffects: Following surgery, a medicated mesh gauze is applied to the face over the abraded areas. Moist gauzes, applied over the medicated gauze, are removed in twenty-four hours. The medicated mesh gauze remains on the face seven to ten days until it falls off spontaneously with the crusts formed by the dermabrasion. Some surgeons omit the gauze and apply antibiotic ointments.

You are wise to avoid direct sunlight and excessive heat, cold, or wind for at least four weeks. Cosmetics should be avoided until the skin has resurfaced.

Complications: Milia, the formation of pinhead-sized white bumps, develops in about 20 percent of dermabrasion patients. These bumps are not serious and are easily removed. Some degree of pigmentary alteration occurs in all patients. Reduction in pigment is generally temporary; increased pigment may be more persistent, and can be aggravated by too early or too much exposure to the sun. Sunscreening lotions and avoidance of sun are essential for several months postoperatively. Bacterial infections of the skin can be handled with antibiotics if they occur. Viral infections (herpes) are also a possibility and must be treated medically. Hypertrophic scars or keloids (overgrown scars) are rare.

Cost: $500–$1,500.

Scar Revision

Purpose: To substitute a cosmetically acceptable scar for a scar that is already present.

Overview: Every wound that penetrates the inner layer of the skin (dermis) leaves a scar. A cosmetically unacceptable scar is one that is highly visible, heavy, discolored, and even disabling. This can be corrected, but it is a popular misconception that a cosmetic surgeon can eliminate a scar. The complete removal of a scar is not possible. It is most important that anyone considering scar-revision surgery understand this point.

Normal scars mature over a period of one year to eighteen months. During this time they become less red, less thick, less prominent, and softer in consistency. A scar generally looks worst between two weeks and two months after the scar-producing injury, and many people seek correction during this period. Yet, revision of an immature scar yields a less than optimal result and deprives the individual of those benefits derived simply from waiting for the scar to mature. In children, scar correction should be delayed as long as possible and should

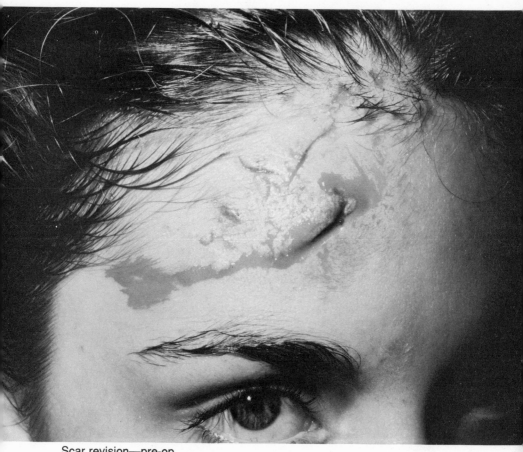

Scar revision—pre-op

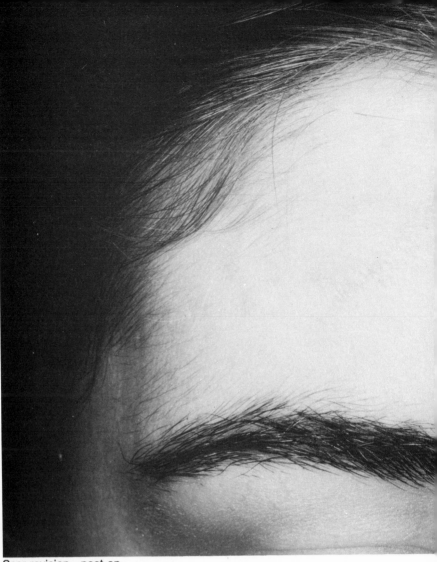

Scar revision—post-op

be undertaken before the scar matures only if it is interfering with some normal function.

Scars that cross body creases caused by flexion tend to widen and thicken. This widening and thickening may occur where there is considerable motion, such as at the cheek-chin junction, the knees, elbows, or shoulders. The injury sustained and the quality of the skin also determine the quality of the scar. The abundant elastic elements in the skin of young children tend to cause scars

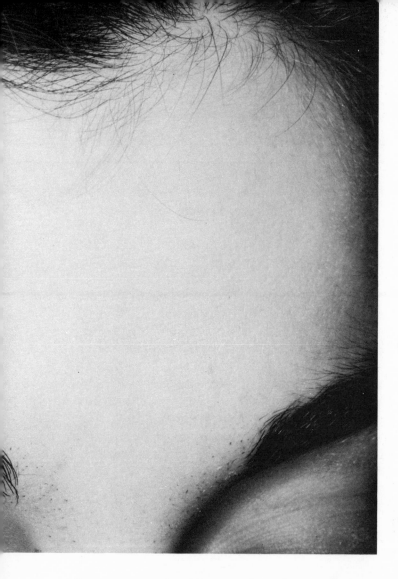

that gape and widen at the edges, whereas the loose, wrinkled skin of the elderly can easily hide scars. Some scars are to all practical purposes invisible; for example, scars on the palms, the soles of the feet, the red portion of the lips, or the inside of the mouth. Scars on the eyelids tend to heal well, whereas scars on the nose may not.

Time and Place: Most scar revisions can be performed in a well-equipped office, although they may be done in a hospital. Local or general anesthesia can be used. The time of the operation varies with the size and shape of the scar to be corrected.

Preparation: An antiseptic scrub (Betadine® or Phisohex®) will be used on the area prior to surgery.

Procedure: Several techniques for correcting scars, ranging from simple excision to Z-plasty or W-plasty, are available. If the scar is crossing perpendicular to the flexion crease, changing the direction of the scar is advantageous. This is best accomplished by a Z-plasty, which changes the direction of the scar and relieves tension along the suture line. The drawback to this procedure is the fact that it lengthens the scar. Vertical scars on the forehead or horizontal check scars often lend themselves to W-plasty correction. The sawtooth excision and its healing characteristics tend to produce a favorable cosmetic result.

Complications: Wound infection as a consequence of hematoma (bleeding under the skin) with subsequent loss of skin is a possible complication. Scar hypertrophy and even keloid (thick scar) formation is a consideration, particularly in black patients. Uneven levels and spreading of the scar can also occur. Dermabrasion may enhance the healing of the scar.

Cost: This depends entirely on the length of the scar and the time it takes to perform the procedure. The price range is $750–$4,000.

Index